Toenail Fungus

The Easy Way to a Toenail Fungus-free Life

(The Treatment and Cure of Toe Nail and Fingernail Fungus)

Walter Rosales

Published By **Jordan Levy**

Walter Rosales

Toenail Fungus: The Easy Way to a Toenail Fungus-free Life (The Treatment and Cure of Toe Nail and Fingernail Fungus)

ISBN   978-1-77485-470-9

No part of this guidebook shall be reproduced in any form without permission in writing from the publisher except in the case of brief quotations embodied in critical articles or reviews.

Legal & Disclaimer

The information contained in this ebook is not designed to replace or take the place of any form of medicine or professional medical advice. The information in this ebook has been provided for educational & entertainment purposes only.

The information contained in this book has been compiled from sources deemed reliable, and it is accurate to the best of the Author's knowledge; however, the Author cannot guarantee its accuracy and validity and cannot be held liable for any errors or omissions. Changes are periodically made to this book. You must consult your doctor or get professional medical advice before using any of the suggested remedies, techniques, or information in this book.

Upon using the information contained in this book, you agree to hold harmless the Author from and against any damages, costs, and

TABLE OF CONTENTS

Introduction

Many people are unaware of being affected by nail fungus. Indeed, many studies suggest that it is one of the conditions that people are prone to overlook particularly when things go towards the worse. For instance, many suffering from yellowing and powdery toenails from fungal infection confess to wearing thick socks to disguise their problem. Many people try to hide their the damaged nails beneath synthetic nails. However, this can make problems even worse.

Many are even misled into thinking that this disorder will eventually disappear by itself. This is the reason why many cases go undiagnosed and untreated for many years.

Many (an estimated one-in-ten) affected by this condition typically have any awareness of their afflicted hands that will eventually become infected. They let these to grow for a long time and can lead to total or partial loss of the nails altogether or, even more serious, the partial or total loss of movement in fingers and toes.

Senior citizens are particularly vulnerable to this disease because of the absence (or insufficient) foot/nail treatment, or as a result of complications from existing medical ailments.

The fact is that having nail fungus is an indication of a microbial problem. In the absence of treatment, it could cause inflammation and infection. This could result in chronic pain, the destruction of the nails (and surrounding tissues and skin) and the loss of mobility of fingers and toes as a result of the scarring or tissue damage.

Additionally, it lowers the body's immune system which increases the likelihood of developing deadly, life-threatening communicable illnesses.

This book gives a broad outline of what nail fungus actually is and the ease to get it. It provides information on who is more likely to contract it, as well as possible complications in cases that are not treated.

This book also includes simple , yet effective preventive measures, as well as solutions at home to treat (or at the very least, reduce signs of) nail fungus and infections. In addition, it offers general guidelines on treatment of hands and feet, and tips on how to improve your the condition of your skin by using "food to treat."

Chapter One: What is Toenail Fungus?

You've likely seen on TV or Internet ads for prescription or over-the-counter medications to treat fungus of the toenail. The ads are targeted to the 35 million people living in the U.S. that suffer from toenail fungus issues. If you've ever had the unpleasing experience of watching commercials, then you're aware that fungus in the toenails doesn't provide a beautiful image. The toenails affected in commercials appear brown or yellow rather than a beautiful pink. Toenails can be deformed and appear extremely thick yet they're brittle. The ugly images could make you believe that hygiene issues are the reason for the toenail fungus. However, it's not true. Even people with impeccable personal hygiene may be victims of toenail fungus.

When the nail bed is in contact with and is infected by a fungal organism it can result in an infection caused by fungal bacteria in the nail. The three primary types of organisms responsible for toenail inflammation are dermatophytes yeasts, and non-dermatophyte moulds.

The majority of fungal toenails and conditions result from dermatophytes that feed on keratin which is the principal nail protein. Also the keratin that is present inside your toenails can be an appealing treat for dermatophytes! In order to compensate the nails begin to make more keratin. They they become so thick they become separated away from their skin. The medical term used to describe toenail fungus is called onychomycosis as well as tinea unguium.For reasons of simplicity in this publication the generic terms of toenail fungus as well as toenail infections are used.

The kind of fungal organism which cause toenail fungus thrives in moist, warm atmosphere. Common locations for fungi that cause infection include footwear that is damp due to sweaty feet, towels that are damp and are tossed onto the ground, showers for public use and gym locker rooms spas, nail salons areas of swimming pools and hot tubs.

If left untreated, a toenail fungus infections can interfere with your quality of life. Senior citizens, in particular are prone to difficulty walking when they have a serious toenail infection. Because of the stigma associated to the condition and to prevent getting the virus, people who are infected may quit walking barefoot. This could mean they will not participate in activities like walking along the beach, attending dance classes or yoga classes or playing activities where shower facilities are common. Your quality of life could certainly be affected by the toenail fungus.

Who is at risk for Toenail Fungus Infections?

Naturally, when preventive measures are implemented when you are in a fungi-rich area reduces the chance of contracting a toenail-fungus infection. There is a chance that you could have a chance of getting it if always wear footwear that doesn't allow air circulate around your feet or if you sweat a lot and you do not alter your shoes at least every other every day, or more frequently in the event of sweating during a workout or sports session.

The best method to ensure prevention from fungus is to ensure that your feet, socks and shoes dry and clean. The use of shoes that do not have a tight fit, are comprised of breathable materials and that are ventilated, can aid in preventing the growth of fungus. This is also the case when using natural cotton socks instead of socks made of synthetic materials that can cause your feet to sweat heavily. It is not the case if you wear socks made of synthetic materials that are specifically designed to draw sweat away from your feet. They are typically available in sports stores as well as outdoor stores (for those who hike). If you wear pants or tights for work it's a good idea to take them off at the end of work, and let your skin breathe.

Toenail fungus is a problem that can affect people of people of all ages, yet it's not typical for children to be affected. Between 25 and 40 percent of people who are older than 60 suffer from fungus of the toes. The likelihood for women is higher develop infections to the toenails than males. This could be because ladies are more likely get regular manicures at spas and salons as opposed to men. Salons and spas may be the first sign of nail fungus infections.

Patients suffering from chronic illnesses such as diabetes or immune-deficiency are at risk of developing foot fungal infections. People who sweat excessively are at risk and can make them more susceptible to infections caused by fungus in the event that they do not maintain the feet clean and wash their their footwear frequently.

If you shower frequently in public areas like the gym or public pool, you could be at greater risk of developing toenail fungus, especially even if you don't use shower shoes and flip-flops.Nail salons are known to be places for nail infections to thrive when dirty towels and soak bins as well as nail tools and other tools are used by several customers and not properly cleaned. Make sure you use only disinfected and clean towels. tools and equipment are utilized during a manicure.

Over 60 years old are also more susceptible to infections of the toenail. Maintaining your feet is crucial regardless of age, but as your body gets older and feet become less healthy, foot care becomes much more crucial. The proper care to prevent fungus includes exfoliation for dead, dry skin, trimming the toenails in a short manner without damaging or cutting your nail bed. Also, gently pressing down the cuticles. Every tool used at home are to be cleaned after every use.

Anyone who wears the socks or shoes of someone with an infection are likely to get an infection. Fungal nail infections are transmissible with an incubation time of 3 to 6 days. If one of your toes is affected and the next toes follow suit, however it's not typical for all toes to become infected. If you've had an infection, unless your footwear you were wearing during the illness are completely cleaned and cleaned, you should dispose of them. If the fungi persist in your shoes you'll be suffering from recurring infections and will lose the fight.

Signs and symptoms of Toenail Fungus

Even if you take the necessary precautions and take care, you could be afflicted with a nail infection with a fungus. There's there is no way to totally stay clear of the bacteria responsible for it. The condition is more apparent over time, however the first indication you may notice are white streaks, or spots on your toenail. It is important to note that streaks or white spots don't always mean toenail fungus. Vitamin and mineral deficiency, allergic reactions to products like nail polish, as well as injuries to the nail may result in streaks of white or black spots on your toenails. It's recommended to have your physician confirm that are suffering from a fungus in your toenails before beginning treatment for it, in the event that you choose to use a natural remedy that will not adversely impact your health or wellbeing.

If you suffer from a toenail fungus the nail can become more thicker and begin to change color. The pale pinkish tone will change to yellowing nails or, in some instances the nail may turn brownish. If the problem persists untreated, and it continues to grow larger, it may be black, and eventually disappear. In most cases, a sour scent can accompany the infection however, it is not always.

The good news is that the disease does not need to progress to the point of affecting the quality of your life or even the losing of the toenail. As you'll see in the following sections of this book, there are natural remedies that work to treat and eliminate the fungus that causes your toenails to grow without needing to use harsh chemicals or drugs that carry a variety of adverse effects warnings.

Diagnosis

With the abundance of medical information accessible on the Internet People tend to diagnose themselves whenever they notice a change in any way to their bodies. This can be the case with changes to the toenails. The self-diagnosis process can be difficult even if you believe you've got all the traditional symptoms of a toenail-fungus disease. There are a few health problems which may be a sign of toenail fungus however aren't. If you're treating toenail fungus while you are suffering from another illness or condition, the second one, that could have a more significant impact, might remain untreated. This is why it is recommended to consult a physician in the event that you suspect toenail fungus. Let the doctor give you an exact diagnosis. When you visit your doctor an in-person sample will be taken and then sent to a laboratory. The report from the lab will show whether you suffer from a toenail infection caused by fungus or another issue.

medical issues that initially seem to be due to a toenail fungus infections can be serious like skin cancer. The first indication of melanoma can be a dark or brown streak beneath the toenail. If the toenails are large and dark this could indicate

Psoriasis. If the toenails show white spots, and they are pitted, alopecia areata may be the issue, not toenail fungus. White and red streaks on the toenails might be signs of Darier disease that is a rare condition.

The difference is between Toenail Fungus is the difference between it and Athletes Foot

When you first realize that you're suffering from foot fungus, it is crucial to identify whether or not it's toenail fungus or athletes foot you're suffering from because both have similarities and distinctions with respect to their symptoms and causes.

Both of them are an infection by fungus that affects the feet, which develop and thrive in moist conditions like running shoes. which is easily transmitted and spread to other areas of the foot but also to others who are in public spaces, like swimming pools, saunas, and the locker room are shared.

Although the causes are very alike, the symptoms the conditions cause are remarkably different. The ailment is triggered by the upper layer of the skin of the feet, whereas toenail fungus is found in the base of the nail. A typical symptom is for feet to be irritated and burned as well as crack, flake and peel, in contrast to the toenail fungus in which the nail changes to a brownish yellow appearance and becomes thicker, breaking up and splitting from the skin during the process.

It's also important to note it is true that the condition known as athletes foot not treated, can result in the fungus that causes toenails. However, toenail fungus does not grow into athletes foot.

Chapter 2: Fungi And Human Nails

The existence of fungi has been around since the time of life's explosion. Man came into existence much later in the biosphere. In the end the two species met and formed an symbiotic connection that is sometimes advantageous to both parties but sometimes detrimental for one or both.

Despite the passing of millennia the fungi have remained at their very simplest form. They have managed to conquer new territories, including living hosts such as Man or, more specifically, certain body parts that are scattered around including genitals, armpits as well as scalps, fingernails, and toenails.

In reality, fungi are present inside and on the outside of the human body but only in tiny amounts make them less dangerous. In conditions that are not ideal there is a chance that fungi multiply in large quantities and cause inflammation, infection and permanent tissue damage.

What exactly is nail fungus?

Nail fungus can be described as an umbrella term that refers to a variety of harmful microorganisms which specifically affect or infect human fingernails and toenails. They include:

* Candida is a genus of invading yeasts that cause the majority of fungal infections that affect Man. There are a few amounts in humans, but are innocuous if the host is generally healthy.

Candida albicans for instance is usually located in the mucous membranes of the human gastrointestinal as well as respiratory system. They are also abundant in the reproductive system of females as well.

They can also be invasive after they have discovered any injury to the skin tissues, especially in the intertriginous area (damaged skin from the constant friction that occurs between the armpits and thighs,) open wounds (including ulcers, lesions, sores, etc.,) or skin always exposed to water.

When the Candida yeast is more virulent and begins to appear in large amounts into the blood, the individual's immunity will be compromised. It opens the way for other pathogens with invasive properties to infect, resulting in the body to become poisoned - the condition known as candidiasis that is systemic.

* Dermatophytes - are the hosts of Ascomycota fungi (over 64,000 species that reproduce sexually) that are most often responsible for triggering inflammation in the keratinized regions in the body of a person, primarily the nails, hair, and the skin. They thrive on Keratin (fibrous structural proteins) and, sometimes, smaller regions with thickened skin (e.g. the skin around nails). Dermatophytes can cause localized pain and swelling.

If they infest areas of skin, they are classified as dermatophytosis, ringworms, or dermatophy. They trigger infections that result in the appearance of a circular or red itchy rash. Ringworms can be extremely itchy and the affected areas develop a thick, scaly and thick skin. In the extreme there's a noticeable loss of hair on the affected region.

If dermatophytes are found in nails, it is referred to as nail fungal infections or dermatophytic ONYCHOMYCOSIS, or simply onychomycosis. This causes a myriad of irregularities in nails. In the worst instances, nails can disappear permanently and the surrounding tissues may become very infected, too.

There are many kinds of dermatophytes. Many of which are already inhibiting specific parts in the body. However, the fungi could easily transfer its seeds and spores from one part of the body to another. This includes:

OEpidermophyton floccosum

oMicrosporum gypseum

oTrichophyton interdigitale

oTrichophyton rubum (most present in the body of the individual)

oTrichophyton soudanese

OTrichophyton tonsurans and

oTrichophyton violaceum

* Tinea is part of the dermatophyte group, and causes similar harm to the human body in infections, with the exception that they

17

don't reproduce sexually. The microorganisms multiply through fission (one cell splitting two smaller organisms or clones) or budding (one portion of the cell is broken off to form a distinct or smaller clone like organism).

They can also transfer their clones or buds from one body part to the next in the course of an infestation. They include:

oTinea unguium - infects nail(s)

OTinea capitis is a scalp infection, a.k.a ringworm of the hair, also known as scalp ringworm

OTinea corporis is seen all across the body, however, it is commonly found on legs and arms

OTinea Cruris - affects the groin a.k.a. jock itch or the groin, a.k.a. ringworm.

OTinea faciei it infects the skin of the face, or even the entire head

OTinea manuum can be found in hand(s) hand(s). While it has the same symptoms as athletes' foot however, this microbe is more potent and can be transmitted to a host via sexual contact even though there is no obvious sign of it.

OTinea nigra infection causes the affected area to become darker in hue

OTinea pedis is a foot/feet infection also known as athlete's foot

OTinea versicolor the infection causes affected areas to discolor and result in skin patches that vary in shades of darkness or the appearance of redness.

So, the most frequent nail fungi that cause permanent or lasting damage to nails are dermatophytic onychomycosis as well as tinea Unguium. The fungi affect fingernails as well as the toenails. However, it is more prevalent with the toenails. According to a study from 2013, one of ten adult people across North America suffers from this disease, and half patients are not diagnosed and/or treated even when they are chronically inflamed, causing repeated periods of discomfort.

This is an extremely risky procedure that seriously weakens the person's immune system, thus increasing the likelihood of developing various life-threatening medical conditions.

Who is at risk?

Men are more at risk of contracting nail fungus and it is most often observed in older men than teenagers or children younger than 12 years old.

Seniors are particularly vulnerable to this disease due to the poor circulation of blood and due to the fact that nails become thinner but larger as they the passage of time. A lot of geriatric patients also suffer from medical conditions which can make the situation more difficult. Certain cases are caused by insufficient or inadequate foot and nail health.

Although it isn't an infectious or contagious condition one can get it if they is living in close proximity to family members or friends who have already been diagnosed with nail fungus, or are prone to regularly or frequently develop one or more types of yeast or fungal infections.

They also have a higher chance of getting this infection if:

* Consistently have poor hand, foot and nails hygiene (or general hygiene issues)

Wearing artificial nails for a long time or subject their nails to excessive embellishments or embellishments.

* Suffer from any nail infection or injury or near the nails.

Have you got infected nails

There is a buildup of moisture in the fingers and toes (or generally, on the hands or feet) for long durations of time

* Also have other types of active infections that are caused by maceration (or break-up of the or breakdown of) or the intertigo (reddening as well as irritation to the skin because of friction or skin rubs painfully against one the other)

* Live or work in unsanitary areas for long durations of time

* Don't smoke, as smoking causes blood circulation to be compromised and causes nail damage on their own

* Do not swim in public pools Unclean or untreated swimming pools

* Do not swim in dirty or unsafe areas of the water (e.g. water bodies that are contaminated, such as marshlands, ponds, wetlands, etc.)

* Are prone to sweating often, particularly those who live in hot, but humid climate.

• Avoid using unsanitary nail cleansing tools and equipment or visit nail salons that do not wash and disinfect their equipment effectively

* Wade through or a long bathing in unsanitary water (e.g. shower rooms for communal use and flood water, public toilets, street puddles, etc.)

* Wear closed-toe footwear (e.g. rubber shoes, boots, e.g.) and socks (that hinder the circulation of nail and the skin, and are not water repellent) for extended durations of time

• Wear gloves that are not properly fitted especially those that hinder normal circulation to fingers and wrists;

* Wear wet or liquid-absorbent gloves during prolonged durations of time

Don't wear shoes that fit poorly and shoes that are tight, especially ones that stop blood flow to your toes. Shoes that are loose could be equally harmful, since the toes are naturally inclined to grasp as much area as possible to hold the body upright. This creates greater pressure and strain on the toes and thereby restricting blood flow to the nails.

People with medical conditions can also be prone to nail fungus, especially those with

* Immune system that is compromised This includes:

OAsplenia (absence of spleen function,) as well as hyposplenia (severely reduced spleen function)

OAgammaglobulinemia (the body does not produce antibodies)

oHave candidiasis

If you have a compromised immune system, it could be because of a recent illness or an operation that was recently major in scope

oHypogammglobulinemia (decrease in production of one or more types of antibodies)

OT-cell deficiency, typically an oT-cell deficiency that is caused by the beginning in...

SSHuman ImmunodeficiencyVirus (HIV) or

SSAcquired Immune Deficiency Syndrome (AIDS)

* Conditions that can affect the circulatory system especially:

OAneurysms or blood clots (in any area within the body)

Arteriosclerosis, oArteriolosclerosis and/or atherosclerosis

oCardiomyopathy

OCoronary heart disease

ODiabetes

Type I diabetes SSType

SSType II diabetes

SSGestational diabetic (temporary blood glucose or an imbalance in insulin due to pregnancy)

SSGeriatric diabetes (blood glucose or insulin imbalance due to the ageing process and further complicated by medical ailments)

OHypertension and stroke

OMyocarditis and Pericarditis

Obesity, or being overweight

O Peripheral Artery Diseases (PAD)

ORaynaud's disease (small and narrowed arteries that are located in the ears, extremities, lips, nipples or nose)

OVaricose veins, or veins that are enlarged due to valve problems

OVasculitis (inflammation of blood vessels)

* Conditions that affect the integumentary organs, in particular:

Abscess complications

Complications of carbuncle

OComplications of Lupus

Complications of necrotizing fasciitis

oDecubitus ulcer (bed sores)

Oeczema (Dyshidrotic as well as Seborrheic)

oErysipelas

OPSoriasis is an incurable condition that affects the skin. It can take it's form as erythrodermic plaque, guttate, and pustular

oStatis dermatitis

Chapter 3: Toe Fungus: An Overview

The idea of having toenail fungus can cause some people to shiver. It's not obvious today however, it is estimated that there will be millions infections of the toenail throughout the United States alone every single year.

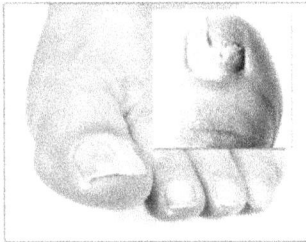

More than three million new cases develop within the United States, making this condition among the most frequent ailments that affect the populace.

The result is a sloppy nail or a nail set. Infected people may notice an abnormal growth in their nails, cracked or chipped toenails, or toenails that are discolored.

In reality, the symptoms are quite common and while it is possible to see a doctor to determine whether you are suffering from it but you are able to determine the condition at your home.

The circumstances are clear:

Brittle toenails

Cracked or dry toenails

Unattractive toenails

Unusual growth of the nails or an abnormal nail growth

Nails that are discolored

Many toenails affected at the same time

There is only one infected toenail at one time

The smell of feet

It could be pain on the nail or inside the toe the toe itself

As you can see from these guidelines, it's simple to determine whether you're suffering from the condition. If you're not sure and really need advice from a specialist and you're not sure, then visit the doctor but remember that this isn't necessarily a risky condition It's just something that requires treatment once you recognize you have it.

A lot of people in the world today don't even realize they suffer from toenail fungus. It is possible to feel discomfort however, generally speaking, toenail fungus can be a unaffected condition that is only resulting in poor health for the toenails. It can spread to other nail beds, and can even spread between people when there is the proper contact.

What that means is that you could be a victim not just by your own circumstances and surroundings, but be able to catch it from things like gyms, the public pool, and even when you try on shoes in department stores.

Of of course there are a number of steps you can adopt to ensure that you don't get this at all We're going to look at them first. Then, we'll explore other reasons and the best ways to treat them.

First , the best way to protect yourself while out and out is to wear socks and shoes

If you find yourself in an area where you have the feet of your shoes exposed be sure that you wash your feet thoroughly using hotsoapy water and then dry them completely once you're done

Do not try on shoes of other people or socks

Avoid wearing shoes that do not have socks regardless of the location

Make sure to change socks once you've tried them on and wash them promptly

Always clean your feet following you've worn shoes, regardless of the location or what you were wearing when you tried them on.

Always follow the safest route regardless of the location or with whom you are with.

As I've mentioned that the world is flooded with millions of cases of toenail fungal infection each year. The greater the exposure you make to outside world and the more exposed you will be exposed to the disease.

However there are many out there who may not even be aware they're infected and, as a result, they're spreading the infection to everyone in the vicinity without knowing that they're doing it.

This is the reason you have to be sure to take every precaution to safeguard your feet and yourself while you're out and about around the globe. The more you take precautions the greater chances you have of being able to avoid recurrence of the fungus.

This is only a brief overview. It is important to know how you can take care of the nail, and also how to prevent the same thing from happening once more.

Don't worry. In the next chapter we'll examine ways to manage this condition completely at home and also what could you do prevent from recurring in the future.

All-round success There's anything better than treating your health issues at home!

Chapter 4: Signs and symptoms and Complications

Fungi usually thrive in moist and warm conditions. This allows them to grow faster which allows the buds or seeds to multiply with no restriction. Although it is not visible to the naked eyes A single fungus reproduces (via sexual reproduction) and reproduces (via the process of asexual reproduction, also known as by cloning) itself from 25 to 100 times over just several hours. Every bud or seed performs the same when it becomes sexually mature, a process which takes only several days, at the very minimum.

This makes it simple for any harmful fungus to infect a nail or an area of skin within a very short amount of time.

However, when a particular body part or area gets over-populated by these microscopic invaders their seeds and buds are able to drop anyplace and drop anywhere. They may land on a different area of skin, nail or even the body part. If they find the perfect setting, the flowers and seeds will invest almost all their energy into developing quickly, and then begin the replication and reproduction process throughout.

This is the reason many people develop nail fungus that affects one fingernail or toenail first, and then the remaining fingernails eventually develop the infection too. The infection can also cause damage to the tissue and skin.

If the seeds and fungi buds are unable to find suitable habitats or hosts, they drop onto the ground or on any other surface. They are able to stay dormant for many years appearing dead in any dry surface. They move unconsciously due to the action of wind or through the movement of humans or animals and allow fungi to locate the right hosts with minimal effort. Just a little bit of rubbing or rubbing the furniture the floor could cause dormant fungi buds to pop and seeds flying in the air.

When the perfect environment has been discovered, fungi can resume their original task of multiplying.

This is the way that this disease can be passed on between people the next (especially in the case of sharing rooms or engage in frequent lengthy interactions) even though nail fungus does not transmit in nature.

What to be aware of

Signs that nail fungus is present and nail fungal infections include:

• Disfiguration or abnormal growth or growth abnormally nail(s), e.g. strangely shaped or bent nail(s);

* Blisters around and near the nail(s) is a normal negative reaction in the case of fungal infections.

* Crumbling and crumbling corners and the tips on the nail(s) that make the appearance of ragged, uneven and uneven. This condition is called distalonychomycosis.

* Lines, bumps, and ridges that appear on surfaces of nail(s) usually discolored or uneven

The buildup of debris underneath the nail(s) could occasionally emit an unpleasant odor

* Coloration of nail(s) because different fungi can appear in various shades

* Dull-looking nail(s) or in extreme instances dead, blackened or dead nail(s)

The flaky nail(s) and the skin around the affected region. This can cause swelling of the flesh that lies directly beneath the nail(s) which is known as subungual hyperkeratosis.

* Nail(s) breaking easily, causing them break and split.

* Nail(s) separating from the flesh, which causes them to break off

Odor that emanates from the afflicted nail(s)

* A powdery or soft nail surface

* Pus that forms under the nail(s)

* Swelling or reddening of the skin around the nails(s)

* Sensitivity or tenderness of the flesh surrounding and under the nails(s)

The thickening process of nail(s) in areas that are uneven or in layers

* Dots of yellow or white appearing on and/or beneath the nail(s)

* Yellow or white streaks that appear in the bottom of nail(s) is a condition known as proximal onychomycosis.

* Yellow or white streaks that appear in the nail bed(s) or under the nail(s) This condition is known as Onychomycosis lateral

In extreme instances chronic pain may be experienced when the fingers or the toes are touched or the pressure of a hand (e.g. taking things off) or toes (e.g. while walking)

These symptoms do not appear simultaneously however, obviously. If the condition is mild, just some of the indications and signs of nail fungus are observed, if any (e.g. there is no discoloration of the nails however there is an odor that is faint from the affected finger).

Advanced cases show a variety of symptoms and signs, which are further aggravated by the patient's slow healing ability, poor care of feet or nails or medical issues.

Untreated and undiagnosed nail fungus can cause unattractive nails, which increases the chance of developing health issues as a result of infections, blood poisoning and harmful microbial infections.

It can also make it difficult to manage current medical issues, for example:

* Chlamydia is an STD or sexually transmitted infection. STD

* Common cold

* Conjunctivitis or more often referred to as pink eye

Genital herpes, warts, or human papillomavirus or HPV, STDs in all forms.

* Giardiasis (a water-borne illness that encourages parasitic infection)

* Gonorrhea, STD

* Hand foot, mouth and hand disease

* Hantavirus Pulmonary Syndrome or HPS

* Hepatitis, a virus infection that affects the liver, leading to inflammation of the internal organs

* HIV and AIDS are acquired through unsafe sharing of needles, sexual activity or STD

* Influenza

* Measles

* Methicillin-resistant Staphylococcus Aureus or MRSA (bacterial infection that afflicts the skin)

* Open sores leading to ulcers, and various forms of epidermal and dermal infection (e.g. cellulitis, etc.)

* Pelvic inflammatory disease PID and STD

* Pertussis, more popularly referred to as whopping Cough

* Ringworms

* Shigellosis (a bacteria-related disease that affects the digestive system)

* Strep throat

* Syphilis, STD

* Tuberculosis (an airborne illness)

* Viral gastroenteritis, also known as more commonly referred to as stomach flu

The most severe cases of nail fungus result in chronic discomfort or sensitivity to the affected area. The affected person's mobility is limited and hinder people from regularly using fingers (fingernail fungus) as well as toes (toenail fungal infection.) Any pressure applied to infected fingernails can cause fluid or pus buildup or even destroy the surrounding structures, such as the cuticle, the nail bed, lunula (half-moon crescent located at nail's base,) matrix (nail base or root from which nail growth begins,) and the nail bed (piece of skin that lies directly beneath that nail.)

Chapter 5: Easy Treatment 101: Caring For Your Nails

Now, let's move on to the most enjoyable part to the problem...the solution.

They are tried and tested techniques that are all efficient. It is important to stick in your approach and if you stick to them then you'll achieve the results you're looking for in just a couple of days.

Keep in mind that consistency and perseverance are the best approach.

Apple Cider Vinegar

What you'll need:

Baking soda

Large bowl

A light scrubber or sponge is ideal for your feet

1/4 cupapple cider vinegar

Directions:

In a large dish or bowl that is filled about halfway by warm water. The dish should be large enough to accommodate the foot that is infected inside.

Add the other ingredients and then soak the feet, making sure that the nails are submerged by several inches of water.

Take a bath for about half an hour.

Then, pour the water out of the tub, then take your scrub sponge or sponge and gently scrub your infected toes.

Rinse your body thoroughly using water that is as hot as you can handle Be careful to avoid burning yourself. After you have rinsed thoroughly then sprinkle with a small amount of baking powder, then dry completely.

Let your feet air dry for at minimum another 30 minutes. It is important to make sure that the sole of your shoe is completely dry before covering it once more.

You can sleep with your feet naked.

Do this every day for a few weeks for a couple of weeks, and the problem will be resolved.

White Vinegar

What you'll need:

White vinegar 1/4 cup

Baking soda

Large bowl

A light scrubber or sponge is ideal for your feet

Directions:

In the dish or bowl of a large size you can fill it half by warm water. This dish should be large enough to place the foot infected inside it.

Add the other ingredients and then soak your feet until the nails are submerged by several inches of water.

Soak for about 30 minutes.

Then, pour the water out of the tub. Take your scrub or sponge and gently scrub the affected toes.

Rinse thoroughly with the hot water you can handle Be careful not to burn yourself. After you have rinsed thoroughly then sprinkle with a small amount of baking powder, then dry completely.

Let your feet breathe for at least another half hour. It is important to make sure the foot remains dry prior to covering it once more.

You can sleep with your feet naked.

Repetition these steps daily for about a week and your condition will be resolved.

Tea oil from trees

12 drops of tea tree oil

Baking soda

Large bowl

A light scrubber or sponge is ideal to clean your feet

Directions:

In a large dish or bowl that is filled half of warm water. The dish must be large enough to accommodate the foot that is infected inside it.

Incorporate the other ingredients and then soak the feet, making sure that the nail is completely submerged by several inches of water.

Soak for about 30 minutes.

Then, pour the water out of the tub, then take your scrub or sponge and gently scrub your infected toes.

Rinse your body thoroughly using water that is as hot as you are able to stand however, be sure to avoid burning yourself. After the water has been thoroughly rinsed you can sprinkle a little of baking powder, then dry completely.

Allow your foot to air dry for at minimum another half hour. You should ensure the foot remains completely dry prior to covering it once more.

Doze with your feet in bare feet.

Do this every day for about a week for a couple of weeks, and the problem will improve.

Coconut oil

Baking soda

Large bowl

Light scrubber or sponge for your feet

1/2 cup coconut oil that is fractionated

Directions:

In the dish or bowl of a large size that is filled about halfway by warm water. The dish must be large enough to accommodate the foot that is infected inside it.

Add the other ingredients and soak your feet, making sure that the nails are submerged by several inches of water.

Soak for 30 minutes.

Pour the water out of the tub, then take your scrub sponge or sponge and gently scrub your infected toes.

Rinse thoroughly with water that is as hot as you are able to stand Be careful to avoid burning yourself. After the water has been thoroughly rinsed you can sprinkle a little of baking powder, then dry completely.

Let your feet breathe for at least another 30 minutes. It is important to make sure that the sole of your shoe is completely dry prior to covering it with a second layer of protection.

Doze with your feet in bare feet.

Repetition these steps daily for a few weeks and your condition will be resolved.

Oil of orange lavender

Baking soda

10 drops of orange oil

10 drops of lavender oil

Large bowl

A light scrubber or sponge is ideal for your feet

Directions:

In the dish or bowl of a large size you can fill it half by warm water. The dish must be large enough to accommodate the foot that is infected inside it.

Add the other ingredients and then soak the feet, making sure that the nails are submerged by several inches of water.

Take a bath for about half an hour.

Pour the water out of the tub, then take your scrub or sponge and gently scrub your infected toes.

Rinse your body thoroughly using water that is as hot as you are able to stand however, be sure to ensure you don't burn yourself. After you have rinsed thoroughly you can sprinkle a little of baking powder, then dry completely.

Let your feet breathe for at least another 30 minutes. You should ensure your feet are completely dry prior to covering it once more.

Doze with your feet in bare feet.

Do this every day for about a week and your condition will improve.

Baking soda

1 cup Baking soda per day

Large bowl

A light scrubber or sponge is ideal for your feet

Directions:

In a large dish or bowl you can fill it about halfway by warm water. This dish should be large enough to accommodate the foot that is infected inside it.

Add the other ingredients and then soak the footto ensure that the nails are submerged by several inches of water.

Take a bath for about half an hour.

Then, pour the water out of the tub, then take your scrub or sponge and gently scrub the affected toes.

Rinse with that is as hot as you can stand, but be cautious to ensure you don't burn yourself. After you have rinsed thoroughly then sprinkle with more baking powder, and then dry completely.

Allow your foot to breathe for at least an additional half hour. You should ensure that the sole of your shoe is dry prior to covering it once more.

Doze with your feet in bare feet.

Do this every day for a few weeks and your condition will be resolved.

Oregano oil

Baking soda

15 drops of oregano oil

Large bowl

Light scrubber or sponge for your feet

Directions:

In a large dish or bowl that is filled about halfway of warm water. The dish should be large enough to accommodate the foot that is infected inside it.

Add the other ingredients and then soak your feet, making sure that the nails are submerged by several inches of water.

Soak for 30 minutes.

Then, pour the water out of the tub. Take your scrub sponge or sponge and gently scrub your infected toes.

Rinse thoroughly with water that is as hot as you are able to stand however, be sure to avoid burning yourself. After you have rinsed thoroughly you can sprinkle a little of baking powder, then dry completely.

Let your feet air dry for at minimum an additional half hour. You should ensure that the sole of your shoe is dry before covering it once more.

Doze with your feet in bare feet.

Do this every day for about a week for a couple of weeks, and the problem will be resolved.

Mouthwash for mouths made of Listerine

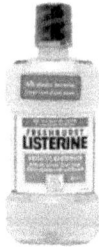

Baking soda

1 measuring cup of mouthwash

Large bowl

Light scrubber or sponge for your feet

Directions:

In the dish or bowl of a large size you can fill it half of warm water. This dish should be large enough to accommodate the foot that is infected inside.

Incorporate the other ingredients and then soak your feet until the nail is completely submerged by several inches of water.

Soak for 30 minutes.

Pour the water out of the tub. Take your scrub sponge or sponge and gently scrub your infected toes.

Rinse thoroughly with water that is as hot as you can handle Be careful to avoid burning yourself. After the water has been thoroughly rinsed you can sprinkle a little of baking powder, then dry completely.

Allow your foot to breathe for at least another 30 minutes. You should ensure your feet are dry prior to covering it once more.

You can sleep with your feet naked.

Do this every day for about a week for a couple of weeks, and the problem will improve.

Olive oil

Baking soda

1/3 cup olive oil

Large bowl

Light scrubber or sponge for your feet

Directions:

In a large dish or bowl you can fill it about halfway of warm water. The dish should be large enough to accommodate the foot that is infected inside it.

Incorporate the other ingredients and then soak your footto ensure that the nails are submerged by several inches of water.

Soak for 30 minutes.

Then, pour the water out of the tub, then take your scrub or sponge and gently scrub the affected toes.

Rinse thoroughly with water that is as hot as you can handle however, be sure to avoid burning yourself. After you have rinsed thoroughly you can sprinkle a little of baking powder, then dry completely.

Allow your foot to breathe for at least an additional half hour. It is important to make sure that the sole of your shoe is completely dry prior to covering it once more.

Doze with your feet in bare feet.

Do this every day for a few weeks and your condition will be resolved.

The Best Blend

Baking soda

10 drops of tea tree oil

12 drops of orange oil

1/2 cup apple cider vinegar

Large bowl

A light scrubber or sponge is ideal for your feet

Directions:

In a large dish or bowl you can fill it half of warm water. The dish should be large enough to accommodate the foot that is infected inside.

Add the other ingredients and then soak the footto ensure that the nails are submerged by several inches of water.

Soak for about half an hour.

Pour the water out of the tub, then take your scrub or sponge and gently scrub your infected toes.

Rinse your body thoroughly using water that is as hot as you can handle however, be sure to avoid burning yourself. After the water has been thoroughly rinsed then sprinkle with a small amount of baking powder, then dry completely.

Let your feet air dry for at minimum another 30 minutes. You should ensure the foot remains dry prior to covering it with a second layer of protection.

You can sleep with your feet naked.

Do this every day for about a week for a couple of weeks, and the problem will improve.

Chapter 6: What is the Cause of Nail Fungus?

The majority of nail fungal infections result from the dermatophyte
fungus. Additionally, yeasts and molds may be the cause. They are the only organisms that are able to thrive in the absence of sunlight.

Certain fungi can be beneficial. But, those which don't require sunlight are found under these conditions:

You can survive in humid, warm conditions, like your bathroom or pool

The fungi can get into your skin through cut-outs, between nails and bed of the nail.

Could cause problems if nails are often exposed to warm, humid conditions.

Nail infection or damage that is early in the process or the skin

You live in a moist or humid climate.

These are only some of the signs that could cause nail fungus, as often the issue appears to appear out of the blue.'

Three Kinds of Nail Fungus

Nail fungus-related problems could be caused by various types of fungi, either in isolation or together:

Dermatophytes

This kind of fungus may be found on hair, skin, or nails. It is the most frequent cause of Athlete's Foot, but it can be a problem for toenails as well. The infection can be contacted through shoes, clothing and shower floors, clippers, or showers and almost any other place the fungus is present. It is the most frequent reason for fungal infections in the toenails.

Yeasts

This kind of fungus may be found on our nails and skin. A yeast overgrowth can be caused by birth control pills, illness or problems with the immune system which could lead to the development of a yeast infection.

Molds

The kind of fungus known as nondermatophytes, or mold, is typically found in soil. It is also able to be found on the skin and nails, but they are typically not transmittable to others.

How To Treat Enail Fungus Is Treatable

A lot of times, nail fungus is identified through its appearance and symptoms. The discoloration may be a sign of other conditions. If you're unsure you are experiencing nail discoloration, it is recommended to conduct a test in a lab done on a sample from the nail.

Chapter 7: What's the Problem with OTC and Prescription Medicine

Prevention is the most effective option with regards to nail fungus. When an infection does occur there are a variety of methods to cure it. The over-the counter treatments are available in liquid or cream form and apply them to the nail mattress and skin surrounding it are available at grocery stores and pharmacies. The topical treatments might help with less severe cases of fungal infection but they're not able to reach the nail bed, therefore their effectiveness is only limited. Although they can be considered to be less harmful than prescription drugs, these treatments may cause adverse consequences, among which the most common is itching, peeling or burning sensations on your skin.

When over-the-counter remedies, many individuals seek out a doctor to get an order for oral antifungal medicine. The prescription treatments are more effective however, the toenail fungus may be recur after the treatment is completed, and the adverse effects of medications are a worry for the majority of people.

The most frequently prescribed nail fungus medicines is Lamisil(tm) it is an antibiotic for antifungal purposes that is recommended to be used for a period of six to twelve weeks. The most frequent side effects for Lamisil(tm) are as follows as diarrhea, stomach upset discomfort in the stomach, nausea nausea, skin rash, headache, and itching. In less common cases, the patient might experience headache as well as a decreased amount of lymphocytes in bloodstream, fever issues with eyesight, and much more. In rare instances, adverse effects could include liver failure that is acute as well as hearing issues, anemia and acute Lupus Superficialis as well as inflammation in the lung. With this list of adverse effects, it is easy to see why some might prefer a treatment which is more natural and less drastic.

Based on Consumer Reports (Reports, 2016) two of the newest nail fungus lacquers available on the market tavaborole (Kerydin(tm)) and efinaconazole (Jublia(tm)) can aid in treating a nail fungus , but are not the most effective. The findings are from studies that show that the drug must be used every day for a period of 11 months, cured fungal infections in 6.5 or 17.8 percent of patients. Based on the report the cost of the medicine was around 600 dollars per bottle!

If you're thinking that there should be more efficient, healthier and less costly ways to treat a fungus-related infection of your toenails You're correct. If you've figured out the treatments you shouldn't apply, let's look at some alternatives.

Chapter 8: Anti Fungal Healing Oils & Herbs

Essential Oils:

There are a variety of important oils as well as carrier oils (the oil mixed with essential oils in order to make it more easily absorbable through the skin) with anti-fungal qualities. If used correctly essential oils can be extremely helpful in the treatment of fungal conditions, and they are healthy, safe and comfortable to apply. Who doesn't like that fresh and clean smell of citrus oil or lavender oil?

Essential oils that fight fungus remove the root of infections in the toenail However, they don't immediately work or even after only a few times. Continue using the oils until sure the issue is removed and your nail is healed. Be patient and you'll notice results in about 8 to 10 weeks, according to the extent of your personal condition of toenail fungus as well as the body's immune system. If you're prone to fungal infection, it's recommended to apply essential oils that fight fungal infections in a lesser frequency to prevent the risk. (A important note: When combating a toenail fungus Avoid using nail polish or any other irritating substances.)

If you are purchasing essential oils, be sure you buy the purest essential oils. If you buy oils that aren't pure, you won't get the benefits of those active components that eliminate fungi. Pure essential oils cost more than blends of chemical-type oils However, remember that a small amount of oil go far Don't be frightened by the cost for tiny bottles. The oils that have antifungal properties and are utilized in the recipes below are on the cheaper end of the spectrum. Essential oils can be purchased at many grocery stores for health, a few pharmacies, and buy them on the internet through various businesses. Make sure you are aware of exactly what you're buying.

Certain essential oils could burn the skin when used in the absence of a carrier oil, or in the case of excessive use and applied cautiously. Like all other medicinal substances that are natural or alternative, make sure that the oil is away from young children. Be sure to not apply the oil to carpets, clothing or furniture because the oil could cause a stain to appear oily. Make sure to apply the oil on dry, clean feet.

Tea Tree Oil

Tea tree oil also known as Melaleuca alternifolia is a great base oil to begin with to fight fungus that causes toenails. It is antifungal in nature and is extremely effective in fighting fungi due to its high content of terpenes. Ideally, to treat fungus on the toenails 70 to 100 percentage tea tree oil must be utilized. Tea tree oil is best used for topically-only. You can dilute it using an oil of a tiny amount like honey or almond oil prior to applying. Soak a cotton-swab in the oil (use the clean swab after the application) and then apply the oil directly onto the toenail, the bed and the skin around it. Repeat the process three times per day.

To add a healing boost by applying the oil directly on the nail or as a preventive measure you could also place some drops of tea tree oils into the warm water in a basin and then soak your feet.

Tea tree oil may be used on its own or in combination with other oils. Combining antifungal oils could prove more efficient than just one oil. Tea tree oil is a great option to use effectively in conjunction with any with the other oils. Don't blend essential oils using water, to make them less potent. Instead, always make use of an oil carrier like coconut oil, olive oil avocado oil sweet almond oil or calendula oil to mention just a few. For a general rule of thumb you should add 10 drops of the essential oil for 1 spoon of oil carrier.

Coconut Oil

It is important to note that coconut oil is an exceptional carrier oil due to its containing the medium-chain fat acid caprylic acid as well as lauric acid which breaks the cells walls Fungi and eliminates them. It can also be utilized to treat fungi by applying it to the toe and letting it sit for minimum 15 minutes, however, it is more effective when it is combined by essential oils.

Thyme Oil

Thymol is an antifungal drug found in thyme oil . It is highly effective in treating fungus of the toenail. Many have reported positive results with Vicks(tm) Vapor Rub as treatment for fungus on the toenails. Thymol is among the major ingredients in the vapor rub, and could be the primary reason for why that the product has been cited as a viable treatment for the fungus of the toenail.

Oil of Oregano

Oregano is a culinary herb oregano which spices our Italian food. However, because it is a source of thymol and carvacrol, it's an incredibly powerful weapon against nail fungus.

Clove Oil

Clove oil can help reduce the discomfort that could be associated with an infection of the toenail It also has Eugenol which is an antifungal drug.

As you can see, there are a variety of antifungal oils that could contribute significantly to the treatment of fungus that affects toenails. If you're susceptible to fungal infections keep these antifungal oil in your medicine cabinet, and use them when you first notice indications of an infection.

Garlic Oil

The advantages of garlic as an natural antibiotic are well-known however, the humble plant is also a fungicide for toenails that are infected. When you mix coconut oil with garlic the fungus isn't given much chance. To create garlic oil, crush and chop several cloves of garlic. Mix with a couple of tablespoons of coconut oil (or olive oil or any other oil carrier) and allow to dry for at least 12 hours. Apply the oil on the affected toenails and the skin around it.

Other essential oils well-known for their antifungal properties you can explore include Lemongrass, Lavender, Cassia, Cinnamon, Geranium, Manuka and Rose Geranium,

Antifungal and Immune-System-Boosting Herbs

Although the majority of the oils discussed in the preceding section of this book are that are derived from plants but there are also other types of plants that are useful in the treatment of fungal diseases. There are a variety of commercial herbal remedies that are available to treat toenail fungal infections. Although this book is geared towards home remedies, if your goal is the most straightforward cure, you should consider formulas that have specific herbs to treat fungal conditions instead of generic formulas that could help support the body in the event of an infection but not specifically treat the disease. Find formulas that include goldenseal, marigold and myrrh.

A treatment plan is not complete without the potent herb properties. dried plants can also be infused with oils or combined together with beeswax and oil to create salves that can be applied to the toes that are infected and the around the skin. Herbs you can take internally can make fantastic teas to drink throughout the day. They can be very effective in treating fungal infections. It is also possible to wash your feet with tea and soak them in tea. If you prepare herbal tea, you shouldn't to throw away the pulp after the tea has brewed. The best option is to wrap damp tea leaves in a tiny piece of cheesecloth or gauze and use it as an application of a poultice to the infected toes.

The herbs listed below are safe. However, as like all medications, whether chemical or natural, consult your physician if you experience any adverse reactions. Many health food stores with bulk herbs will carry the following herbs.

Black Walnut Hulls ~ antifungal

Echinacea ~ Immune system boosting

Cloves ~ antifungal

Chaparral Leaf ~ antifungal

Calendula is healing and antifungal

Goldenseal ~ antifungal

Chapter 9: Aiding the Process Affirming Proper Treatment

I can tell you that when you're suffering from something like this, you'd like it to be gone. You need it to go away now.

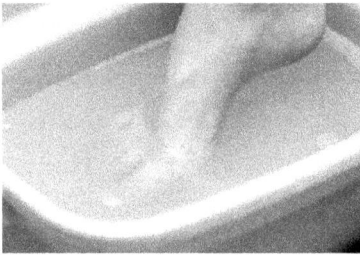

It's more than logical however the reality to the point is that it takes time. For the fungus to go away and heal your toenail it self, you're going to need to work on your nail to ensure it is healing.

That means that you will have to soak your nail in bowls and you should make the effort to do it every single day. Every day that you go by without bathing your foot in the bowls, you're giving fungal growth the chance to multiply and establish itself in your nails again and again.

71

The most important thing to understand about toenail fungus is it's a live thing and it will grow as fast as it is able to.

If you are looking to remove the foot ailment it is necessary to get rid of it. This means that you need to take the time to defeat the enemy.

The fungus was designed to survive in extremely harsh conditions. In order to eradicate it you must demonstrate that you are better prepared and more durable than the fungus. This fungus is alive and is determined to stay on the nail, meaning it's going to endure many treatments before dying.

However If you're conscientious about your treatment, you could find that there is an extremely short amount of time that you need to put on your nail to repair it. It all comes down to perceptions as well as the longer you're willing to spend on your nail, the higher it will be.

However, it is important to keep in mind that you must also make other preparations when you're treating this condition.

The fungus is seeking an ideal place to thrive and the more exposed your nails to spores more likely it will grow in the exact spot it was when it first began.

That is this means that you could be infecting yourself again after having have completed some of the treatment.

Therefore, I would like to make sure that you're making all the necessary precautions required to ensure that you don't put yourself in excessive risk of exposure to this fungus over again. Here's a list items you must take into consideration while you're doing treatment to ensure that you eliminate the fungus completely and do not return it after you're done.

Clean and dry. This is a general rule of thumb that you can follow on all things. Dry and wash the bowl once you're finished, then wash and dry out the bathtub when you dump the water into the tub.

Dry and wash the towel you employ to dry your feet.

Wear gloves. Nails of all kinds can be affected by this fungus and you shouldn't expose your fingernails to the fungus as you attempt to eliminate it from your feet!

Cleanliness is at the top of your checklist.

I'm sure I've said something about doing it twice. But I want to be sure... that fungal fungus isn't a fan of water. It loves moisture however, not water. This means that the longer you leave soap and water on your space when you are cleaning and cleaning, the more likely you'll be able to push it away.

However the more you maintain the area clean in the absence of any direct treatment to you nails, the greater chance the fungus will fade out and never return

It is important to maintain your nails as insidious as you can to the fungus. If you create a space which they aren't able to live in, they're unlikely to attempt. It's all about keeping the advantage in the game and soon after all, you're going to be back on your feet.

Chapter 10: Nail Fungus Treatment

Nail fungus is also known as onychomycosis is a chronic condition that can affect your toenails as well as fingernails.A nail fungus disease is among the "embarrassing" diseases that people tend to avoid discuss about.People are hesitant to speak with medical professionals about their issue, which can frequently delay the treatment.

In the summer, spring and fall months, many of us take part in outdoor activities. It is not unusual to exchange our shoes to wear our favourite sandals.Only the problem is that you've got an infection of your toenail fungus, and you're not comfortable letting everyone look at your ugly toes. It is difficult to wear sandals, or even go without shoes at the beach. Summer and spring become times of worry for those suffering from nail fungus.

Recognizing Nail Fungus Infections

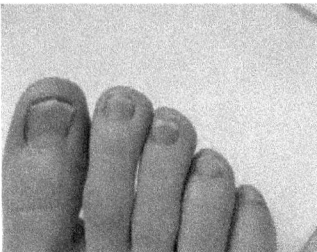

The fungus begins as a white spot at the nail's edge of the patient. The spot grows and makes the nail painful, discolored and forms a rough edge. The discoloration tends to turn yellow over time, which is a great way to distinguish nail fungus from the other ailments.

The nail that is affected by the fungus will become disfigured and rises above regular nail bed. The diagnosis becomes simpler when the distortion is seen on several nails. The nails that have been distorted may become painful due to the shift away off the nail bed.In some instances, the dislocation and dissociation of the bed could cause an unpleasant smell.

Nail Fungus Causes

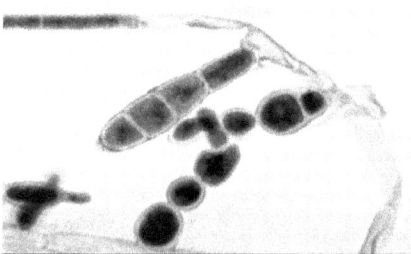

Nail fungal infections result from organisms which are microscopic and called "fungi".They don't require sunlight to flourish and thrive in moist and warm climate. The most prevalent fungi involved in nail problems is classified as Dermatophytes. The most frequent dermatophyte that causes this kind of disease is trichphyton rubrum. There are a variety of other fungi , as well as some molds also are accountable for this condition.

Fungus infiltrates the nail bed which causes nails to become yellow and, eventually, they become sensitive and itchy. The fungus responsible for this type of condition typically thrives in humid and warm environments and is able to find the ideal habitat beneath the nails.The extent of the infection and the severity with which nail fungus has affected can be classified into standard, mild or severe.

Who is a victim of a fungal nail Infection?

A nail fungus can pose an apprehension for victims from all age groups, regardless of their gender or social standing.You know what I mean no matter how much money you earn and your faith or colour of your skin, it is possible to be afflicted with an fungal nail infection.Nail fungal is more prevalent in men than women , and more prevalent among the elderly than those who are young.In fact, nail fungal infections are among the most prevalent diseases of the nails, accounting for around half of all nail problems.

The Contributing Factors that Influence the formation of a nail Fungus

One of the most effective methods to avoid nail fungus infection is being aware of the causes that trigger them, and trying to prevent them.

Inadequate hygiene is the primary risk factor for the development of fungal nail infection.It is caused by the fact that nails are not kept properly clean. It is essential cut your nails regularly and obviously maintain them in a clean state.

Another reason that can cause nail fungus is to wear sweaty and dirty shoes that causes a damp environment around the nails.This allows the fungus to have the perfect environment to thrive and grow, creating an ideal environment for fungal growth to spread and infect the nails.

Sometimes, damage on the nails and the bed can trigger the development of nail fungus. The nail's injuries may cause them to be exposed to fungus, which can infiltrate and occupy the spaces that are created by the trauma.The injury to the nail can be caused by incidents such as hitting the door onto one nail or being hit by something that doesn't create an open wound.The injured nail will usually have dead cells that can create health hazards and creates a perfect setting for fungus to flourish.

If you are prone to sweating a lot, you are more susceptible to fungal infections due the fact that sweating creates an environment that is humid and warm.

Anyone with who have a history of Diabetes and its associated circulation issues will be more susceptible to nail infections.In addition , any medical condition that affects your immune system can cause you to be more susceptible to these kinds of infections.

Shoes that are too tight that cause crowding of your toes could result in nail fungus.Add to this the need for heavy socks that offer little airflow and you've got the ingredients for nail issue.

Nail Fungus Treatment Options

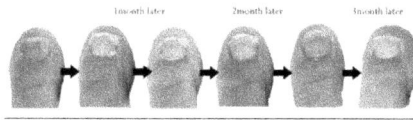

There are many methods for treating nail fungus and all of them claim to different results, which makes it difficult for the majority of people to choose which method is the best for these conditions. The majority of treatments that are available are typically effective, but their effectiveness and time frame of treatment vary. Hence, it is very important to get the most relevant information about the various types of treatments so you can decide which remedy will work best for you given your particular circumstances.Fortunately this infection is treatable for most; however, you need to understand that it takes time for most of the remedies to work.

Home remedies for treating Nail Fungus

Chlorine Foot Bath

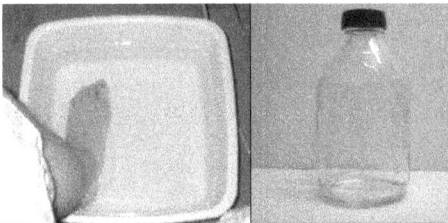

The most sought-after remedies at home is to soak the feet affected in bleach chlorine , which contains one gram of chlorine 10 portions of water. This procedure should be performed at least twice per day, at the beginning of the day and at night prior to going to go to bed. The two sessions will last about 15 minutes. The process should be carried out over a period of two months, at minimum before you begin to see improvements.

Vinegar Foot Bath

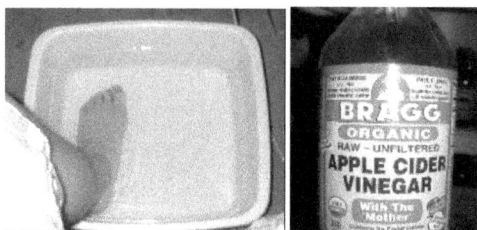

Vinegar dilute by water is often utilized to cure fungal nail problems. Vinegar can combat and eliminate these fungi due to due to its acidity. acidity.Soak your feet in water and vinegar solution each night, and you'll see changes within 3 to 6 months.A variant that is a foot bath made of vinegar composed consisting of one liter of dark beer at ambient temperature, a white vinegar liter and a half-sachet of acidophilus. The feet of the person suffering from the condition are to be bathed in this solution for at minimum 30 minutes per each day for between one and three months. It is essential to keep in mind that feet as well as the nails that are affected must be completely dry after each session to facilitate speedy treatment since the fungi can get worse in moist environments.

Listerine Remedy

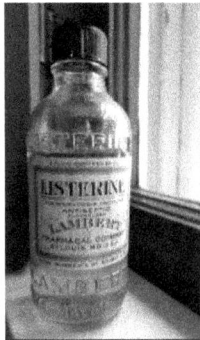

Listerine mouthwash is intended to eliminate oral bacteria. However, it can also to eliminate the fungus that has invaded your nails when you are in certain situations. You can simply soak your affected nails in Listerine at least 10 mins prior sleeping.Continue these soaks at least three months prior to deciding whether the remedy works or not.

Treatment for Nail Fungus

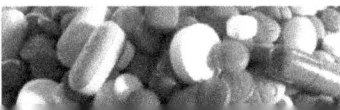

Prescription drugs are frequently employed to treat nail fungus. The medications are prescribed by licensed medical professionals who have the knowledge to recognize which medications will work best. The most commonly used treatments for this condition are Fluconazole, Itraconazole, Lamisil, lopirox, and Amorofine Terbinafine.

These medications typically contain powerful chemical compounds that kill fungal spores by eliminating the fungus which affects the nails. It is essential to exercise caution when taking these medications as some of the stronger chemicals could react negatively to different parts of your body and can cause adverse unwanted side effects. This is particularly true for those suffering from other medical conditions , or who take other medications for treating other conditions. Therefore, it is essential to see a certified medical professional who can determine whether prescribed medications could cause harm to the patient.

Topical anti-fungal treatments are available on prescription rather than taking

the drug orally.These treatments are
applied directly on the nail in the form of a
cream or similar to varnish. These
treatments are thought to can kill the
fungus which causes the infection , but the
penetration through the nail could be
restricted.

Treating Nail Fungus with Vick's Vaporrub

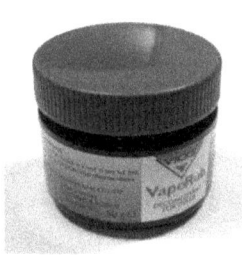

Treating your nails with Vicks Vaporub can
be a natural remedy that appears to be
increasing in popularity.You likely have
heard about Vicks VapoRub can cure
toenail fungus prior to. It's actually a
constituent of Vaporub and thymol (which
is an inorganic derivative of Thyme) that
are believed beneficial in the treatment of
nail fungus.

Researchers have examined the antifungal effect of ingredients found in a generic chest rub. Thymol, one of active ingredients in the medicated chest rubs, was discovered to be effective in inhibiting the development of the dermatophytes which are responsible for nail fungus. Further studies have shown that thyme oil can kill the other cause of nail fungus which is Candida. It does this through disruption of its metabolic cell membranes, as well as its metabolism.

The treatment involves applying Vick's on the affected nail daily.It is advised to ensure that you completely cover the nail, even its base nail.It is suggested to continue this procedure for up to six months.There appears to be a downside to this method is that it could cause mild discoloration to the nail.

A Laser treatment for nail Fungus

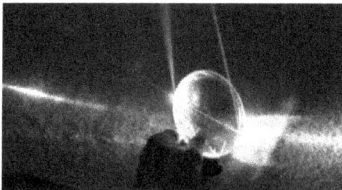

Nail fungus is also treated with lasers that focus laser energy on the affected nail. The laser light enters nails and eliminates the fungus, without harming the skin surrounding. The major benefit of this treatment is that it requires very little time as compared to other treatments. However, the treatment must be performed by an experienced professional as a mistake can cause further harm to the nails. The procedure is expensive as it isn't covered by many insurance firms. Some people believe that the out-of-pocket cost is worthwhile since laser treatments have been shown to be effective in treating the condition within a shorter time.

Nail Fungus

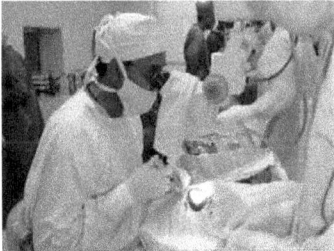

Surgery can also be a treatment alternative for nail fungus. However, I believe it should only be considered as an option last resort. This method of treatment involves surgically eliminating the entire affected nail and thus eliminating the fungal infection. Antifungal creams applied to the skin are typically applied following removal of the nail to stop regrowth while new nails are created. The nail will then grow fresh without infection. The procedure is typically performed by a trained physician who is able to safely remove the nail with no damage to the skin around it. It can take a few years or longer for the nail to heal completely.

Treatment of nail fungus infections

We've heard of the phrase "prevention is worth one pound or cure". It is well-known that fungal infections may be caused by contractions from an individual who is affected by the disease. The fungal infection could spread between one individual to another when there is a channel that allows them to move.

The most obvious way to get a fungal nail infection is to share footwares and socks. The infection can also be spread by sharing other tools like nail clippers cuticle cutters, and other equipment that are used in nail salon.So the main message is to not give away your sneakers, socks or shoes with anyone as you will never be able to tell if they suffer from nail fungus.Make sure that when you go to the nail salon that you bring your own scissors, clippers and other tools regularly employed.

Fungal nail infections can be caused by contact with the fungal fungus within places like the shower floors and locker rooms found at health facilities. It is a good opportunity to maintain a healthy lifestyle and put something on your feet while walking through these places.

In conclusion, it is possible to get rid of nail fungus.What you need to know is that persistence is the best ability in this case in order to eradicate it.Just be aware that it isn't going to disappear overnight, and it may require daily treatment for several weeks or even months. I am mentioning this because I believe it's essential to be aware of all the details before you attempt to treat an incredibly stubborn disease like a nail fungus.

Chapter 11: Viable Home Remedies

There are a variety of solutions at home for toenail fungus that is passed down from generation to generation or published on a variety of websites that are available on Internet. Certain of them have been proven scientifically to be effective, however the majority of them are promoted by people who have had positive experience with the remedy. Here are some natural remedies that you could test.

Garlic

Garlic is an all-around great treatment for a variety of ailments however, several studies have shown that garlic works most effective as an antifungal treatment. Garlic can be consumed as part of a diet plan for maintenance to prevent the growth of fungi however, it is most effective when applied on its own.

Be aware that only fresh garlic needs to be employed in place of capsules or powder.

For garlic to treat fungus on the toenails, put the gauze in a small amount on an uncluttered surface. Add a clove of garlic inside the gauze. Utilizing the back of a spoon, or a knife that is broad, crush your garlic clove. A second gauze sheet should be placed over the garlic that has been crushed. While holding the garlic then place the gauze on your toe. Secure the edges using the adhesive tape of your choice or with an adhesive bandage to ensure it remains in position. Place it on top of your foot for between four and five hours. Remove the bandage , and then repeat the process using clean gauze and an uncut clove of garlic. (Do do not overuse the gauze, or even the garlic clove.)

Antifungal Powder

The antifungal powder was made from an original recipe created by Rosemary Gladstar. The recipe was published in her book Herbal Recipes of Rosemary Gladstar that promote Vibrant Health. The powder of arrowroot and the herbs included in the recipe are usually available in every health store that sells large quantities of herb. In the majority of herbs, the therapeutic properties are contained from the volatile oil found in the plant, so make sure to find the most fresh dry and dried herbs are available.

3/4 cup arrowroot powder

1 teaspoon powdered chaparral

1 tablespoon of powdered black walnut hulls

1 teaspoon goldenseal powdered in powdered form.

1 teaspoon essential tea tree oil from the tea tree

1 tablespoon of oil from oregano

Mix all the ingredients, excluding the oil of tea trees and the oil of oregano in a small dish. Mix the oils well using the help of a fork. Allow the mixture to sit in the bowl, in a dry area where it will not take in moisture for a few hours. Transfer the powder into an airtight shaker bottle or container and keep it in dry place. Sprinkle generously on the affected toe twice a each day as needed.

Antifungal Cream

If you're the DIY kind, this quick antifungal cream recipe could be the answer to your need of relief from fungus that causes toenails. Coconut oil is anti-fungal and soothing. It also helps smooth and soothe the skin that is irritated or thick. Shea butter is available in a wide variety of health food stores where organic products for beauty are available.

Ingredients:

1 cup of coconut oil

1/4 cup beeswax

Shea Butter 1/4 Cup

15 drops of tea essential oil of the tree

5 drops of oil of oregano

Method:

Place the coconut oil in the jar of a quart (Mason or Bell type jars that are used to can.) Add the beeswax and butter to the container. Then, with the lid off, place the jar the lid, in a large saucepan that holds approximately 2 inches of water in it. At a low temperature, heat until the beeswax and the shea butter melts, stirring frequently while taking care not to spill any water into the container. Take the jar off the stove to add the tea tree oils as well as the oil from oregano. Stir until the mixture is well-mixed. Keep the jar in the refrigerator until the mixture has become firm. When the mixture is firm and ready to be taken out of the fridge and allow it to cool at room temperature until it's soft enough to scoop a tiny amount at a stretch to rub onto the toes that are infected.

Vicks VapoRub(tm)

Many have reported relief and the elimination of fungus on their toes by applying Vicks VapoRub(tm) over their toes that are infected. It is commonly used to treat respiratory illnesses and colds, and in vapourizers, the ointment is made up of camphor and thymol, which are considered to be the active ingredients are effective in treating fungal infections.

Homemade Natural Vapor Rub

If you are not able to use any ingredients found in the generic version vapor rub it's easy and fast for you to create your own using all natural ingredients. The recipe is as follows:

1 cup of coconut oil

2 tablespoons of pastilles made from beeswax (found in natural or craft health stores)

18 drops pure eucalyptus essential oil

18 drops pure peppermint essential oil

8 drops of pure essential rosemary oil

10 drops of clove oil

Place butter and coconut oil into an oven-proof pan. Cook on the flame until it is just melting. Take off the heat. Add essential oils. Put the mixture into small jars or tins. Let harden. Rub toes that are affected by the fungus, as required, a few times a day until the the fungus has been eliminated.

Footbaths:

Apple Cider Vinegar, and Baking Soda

While there aren't any evidence to be any studies that show the apple cider vinegar or baking soda foot baths work Many have stated that they have been successful in treating toenail fungus by using the use of baking soda and apple cider vinegar foot soaks. In the simplest terms, the treatment could thoroughly cleanse the feet and soften them as vinegar as well as baking soda are believed to provide healing properties.

Mix equal quantities of vinegar from apple cider and water into an uncluttered basin. Add half to one cup of baking soda. Soak your feet in the foot bath for at least 20 minutes. Dry your feet completely following the soak. Don't reuse the towel until you've washed it. (It's recommended to utilize a white towel which is bleached after every use.) Soak feet in a bathing tub every day for two or three days.

Goldenseal and myrrh footbath

For preparing a footbath made of goldenseal simmer about two to three tablespoons of dried goldenseal in 2 cups of water at a low heat for around 20 minutes to create goldenseal tea. You can strain the tea. Place the tea in a basin that is clean along with an additional cup of water as well as around 10-drops of myrrh-infused tincture. Infuse your feet with the tea. Clean your feet completely using an untidy towel.Repeat at least two to three times a day until the infection has disappeared. Make sure to use a fresh, dry towel to dry your feet.

Chamomile Tea Tree Oil Footbath

Chamomile tea is a great aid in fighting fungus. To make a chamomile-infused tea bath, boil up to three tablespoons of chamomile tea or three tea bags of chamomile in two cups of water on low heat for around 20 minutes. Remove the tea from the strainer or from the bags of tea and put the tea in the basin that is clean. You can add another glass of water, and add 10 drops of tea oil from the tree into the water in the bowl. Soak your feet for around 20 minutes. Dry your feet thoroughly with the use of a clean towel. Repeat this process 2 or 3 times per day until the infection has gone. Always use a dry, clean towel to dry feet.

Listerine(tm) Forefoot Soak

Listerine is renowned for its capability to eliminate bacteria which cause tooth decay however, many people find it useful in eradicating the fungus that causes infections to the nail. To make the Listerine(tm) bath for feet, make use of the amber-colored mouthwash that was originally used. Mix 1 cup Listerine(tm) as well as 1 cup white vinegar into three cups of hot water, placed in a basin that is clean. Soak the feet of your affected for around 20 minutes. Dry your feet completely using an unclean towel after you have soaked the feet. Repeat the process two to three times a day until the infection has gone away.

Chapter 12: Winning the Battle by Keeping Your Nails Yours

It's true...the notion of toenail fungus is disgusting, regardless of the person you are or how many times you've had to deal with it. To make things worse...the possibility of contracting the fungus from another causes the condition to be more serious.

If you've had the experience of getting it and you've experienced it, you're aware of the symptoms, and you definitely don't want to bring it back. If you're not sure of what caused it at all This could be an issue however it is definitely worth getting used to in case you don't want to go through the same treatment once more.

Whatever number of times you've dealt with this issue before If you experience it time and time again, you will have to endure the same treatment over and over again.

If you've faced this kind of treatment prior to, you're aware that it takes some time to address it. This is something you'll be trying to avoid regardless of who you are.

One of the most effective ways to avoid treatment is to stay clear of the issue that needs treatment, which is exactly what we're going to discuss in the next.

It is well-known that toenail fungal infection is widespread and you could become exposed all all over. No matter how well-maintained your feet are, as long as someone sitting next to you is suffering from it, you'll be exposed. It does not matter how much you'd like it not to get under your toes If you're exposed, you're at the risk of being exposed.

This is why we should consider the actions you can do to help to keep this problem at bay. Things you can accomplish in the world that you live in on a daily to day basis will eliminate this issue right from the scene for you. Thankfully. These aren't just easy to accomplish and can help in preventing the disease as the treatment to clear it.

Dry and wash

One thing to follow is that when you're outdoors, you're exposed. Make sure to wash your feet at minimum once every day, and ensure that you're dry!

Do not touch other people or with conditions

You aren't always in control of the situation you're facing, yet if suspect you're in a position that could have led to your being exposed then go back to the initial rule and clean and dry.

You could be exposed and not even realize it, or notice your exposure just as it occurs. In either case clean and dry.

Maintain good hygiene

Don't just clean your feet, clean your socks and clothing or in your shower...anywhere you have your feet exposed.

You're looking to make sure that your surroundings perfect to ensure your foot is safe, and not the fungal growth.

Maintain a good diet

The better you're nails, the more difficult it will be for the fungal growth to take root. Intake plenty of minerals and vitamins, and you'll enjoy many benefits...including your feet!

Clean your feet!

As difficult as it is...the most effective way to combat any kind or infection, is to keep your feet as clean as it is possible. If you make sure your feet are dry and clean, and when you put socks on the shoes you wear, then switch to dry socks after you've finished a sweaty sport, and ensure that your surroundings are foot-friendly then you'll have healthier nails!

The most important thing that I want to remind you of is that anyone can develop toenail fungus. And if you have it, it's not an indication that you're unclean. The most important thing is that you keep it under control and do everything you can to ensure it stays that way.

It is possible to catch it wherever however, the reality is that you can get rid of it similarly, as long as you're determined to keep your home tidy and combat it as it is a mold.

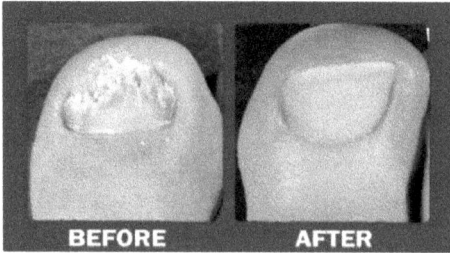

BEFORE   AFTER

Chapter 13: An Overview of the traditional Nail Fungus Treatments

There are many methods to combat nail fungus. In addition to preventive measures, there are also natural remedies as well as topical treatments and oral medicines.

In the traditional Chinese medicine, or TCM, (which has been used for more than two thousand years) nail fungal and fungus infections were treated using the combination of diet therapy, application of a variety of herbal balms, and the use of acupuncture.

Chinese doctors frequently questioned their patients regarding their medical and personal history before presenting any diagnosis. This was due to the belief that whatever activity (including simple chores that are routine, sexual activity, or incident) has always influenced the flow of the chi/qi (sustaining life force for all living things) in the body.

They often suggest small changes to the patient's living conditions for example, drying the feet and hands using a the same cloth after each bath, cleaning the fingernails as well as toenails to remove dirt or soil or vinegar, or using water to bathe the feet or hands or baths for feet, etc.

But, these suggestions were often accompanied by meals which contained food items that were known for their intrinsic healing capabilities. For cases ranging from moderate to severe of fungal nail fungus or nail infection, frequent application of herbal balms, acupuncture and herbal remedies became an element of treatment.

Dietary therapy/Food as therapy

The most commonly used method of treatment for nail fungus during that time was diet therapy (a.k.a. food therapy,) as well as the intake of certain foods to help heal.

Nail fungus is believed to be the result of the gradual decrease in the temperatures of the body's central core (somewhat like chakra.) The thought was that this caused all sorts of ailments that affected the extremities, such as fungal growth on fingernails and toenails.

Thus, food items and drinks that further cool the body (triggered chill energy in or around the yin) were suggested to be cut out of daily meals or, at the very least drinking in a smaller amount.

They include:

* Bamboo shoots

* Banana

* Bitter gourd

* Broccoli

* Cauliflower

* Chrysanthemum tea

* Clams

* Crabs

* Cuttlefish

*Dairy products (e.g. cheese, milk, yogurt, etc.)

Fresh mustard leaves

* Grapefruit

* Lettuce

* Lotus root

* Persimmon

* Salt

* Seaweeds

* Soy sauce

* Star fruit

* Strawberries

* Sweetened and sweetened drinks in particular, those that contain crystals of sugarcane

* Tomatoes

* Water chestnut

* Watermelon

* Bread made of white, especially ones that are made up of barley, buckwheatand wheat and millet

Drinks and food items that cooled the body (triggered the body to release heat or the yin) were suggested to be consumed or included more. They included:

* Abalone

* Apricots, peaches, and nectarines

* Asparagus

* Black coffee

* Chili pepper, black peppers, sweet peppers and Szechuan peppercorns

* Cherry

* Chestnut

* Chicken eggs and chicken.

* Cinnamon

* Coriander

* Dates

*Fennel bulb and frosts

Fresh water shrimps, lobsters, crabs and mussels

* Ginger and garlic

* Glutinous rice

* Goat's milk

* Mustard seeds

* Onions, which include green onions, chives, shallots, and leeks

Pig and Pork liver

* Pomegranate

* Sea cucumber

* Sweet peppers

* Vinegar

* Pine nuts and walnuts

* Wine

Chinese physicians who were practicing traditional medicine typically employ special chefs to cook certain dishes that included "healing" ingredients. So visiting the "clinic" included meals also.

Most of the time the clinics were equipped with pharmacies of their own that offered prepared ingredients (e.g. dried herbs, meat that was cured, etc.) to the general public which can be cooked or eaten at the home.

Doctors will only prescribe herbal balms or Acupuncture in more severe situations.

Herbal balms to treat nail fungus

Common balms for herbs used in traditional Chinese medicine comprised the use of oils and water, for example:

* Alisma helps to reduce inflammation and the symptoms of infections.

* Atractylodis, a.k.a. Cang Zhu, is Rhizome that has as warming properties which purportedly eliminate stomach meridians and spleens. It helps reduce inflammation and swelling, particularly on the extremities.

* Dictamnus, a.k.a. burning bush, is a plant with antiseptic qualities that reduce yeast,

fungal, and bacterial growth in areas of affliction.

* Kochia is a potent antifungal ingredient, and it can be used to treat any kind of Dermatophytes.

* Plantago, a.k.a. plantain leaf, is a powerful antimicrobial properties that eliminate harmful microorganisms such as viruses, bacteria, fungi and yeast.

* Tribulus, a.k.a. puncture vine, is typically used to treat the symptoms of eczema. However, it reduces skin redness and sensitivities, as well as reducing the chances of outbreaks and blisters caused by allergies. fungal infection

Acupuncture

Acupuncture is an old method of inserting needles into specific locations in your body (meridians) to enable the body's life force (chi or Qi) to flow freely without obstruction. The needles are believed to rid these meridians obstructions (e.g. slow or weak blood flow or sluggish blood.) which can cause mental and physical illnesses. Sometimes, these needles can be slightly heated to increase blood flow.

This type of alternative medicine is (and must be) only done by a certified specialist (a acupuncturist who is licensed by the government.)

Modern day home remedies

There isn't a single solution to nail fungus or fungal infections. Different people react differently to different treatment options.

This is why there's many home remedies available. If you have an asymptomatic condition of nail fungus that doesn't experience pain and the problem is restricted to a couple of nails, these remedies for home are suggested.

* Cleansing agents, rubs, soaks, sprays, etc.

OApple cider vinegar is a great source of antibacterial and antimicrobial properties and is able to prevent all sorts of infections.

Make a mixture of apple cider vinegar and equal parts of clean cool water. Put the mixture in an aerosol bottle. Spray affected areas every two to three times per day, or as often as possible. Dry the area thoroughly.

Mix 1/2 cup apple cider vinegar and 2 cups of water that is lukewarm. Soak feet and hands for 20 to 30 mins. Rinse them off lightly. Dry feet or hands thoroughly at the end of each soak. Repeat this process 2 to 3 times per day, or at any time. This can be particularly beneficial in cases where there are more than one nail affected or if hands or feet are also afflicted by other fungal types (e.g. athlete's foot, ringworms, etc.)

Notes: Only do this when there aren't any breaks or splits in nails or skin. Make sure the water isn't too hot to cause further damage to the affected areas. Always create separate soaking solutions for your hands and feet. Avoid reusing soaking solutions.

Alternatives to apple cider vinegar that offer the same healing properties are:

Cane vinegar unsweetened (check the labels before purchasing)

Palm vinegar or Coconut, without sweetener, (check product labels first before purchasing)

SMalt (or sherry vinegar)

Raspberry vinegar

SSWine vinegar, which includes rice wine, as well as white wine vinegars. Red wine can also be used however it can make skin stained, so you should only use it when other vinegars are not available.

OBaking soda, also known as sodium bicarbonate is a great natural deodorant that is helpful for nail infections that are emitting unpleasant odors. It kills the fungi, mold, and microscopic parasites as well.

Applying the powdery substance directly to the face (but not on splits or open sores) can reduce irritation and itching. This is especially helpful for people who might have developed allergies (e.g. blisters, rashes, etc.) due to the presence of fungal infections. Rub gently to remove dead cells with an nail brush. Utilize dry paper towels to remove any debris afterward. Use only when needed.

or dissolve 1/4 cup baking powder in the similar amount of water. Use it to cleanse hands of nail fungus. Dry the area thoroughly afterward. This will make your skin feel soft and more smooth.

You can also prepare a cleanse bath by dissolving 3 TBSPs. in baking soda as well as 3 tablespoons. from apple cider vinegar, in four cups of water that is lukewarm. Soak feet and hands for at least 20 mins. Dry with a towel and air dry afterward. Soak feet or hands daily at least. Other recipes for baths that cleanse include:

SSDissolve three heaping tablespoons. from baking soda, in 1/2 cup of white wine vinegar. Add 2 cups of water.

SSDissolve 3 heaping tablespoons. Of baking soda, in four cups of water that is lukewarm. Pour in the juice of one lime. Add the rinds of a lemon that have been discarded to the liquid that is soaking.

SSDissolve 1/2 cup baking soda as well as 1/2 cup Epsom salt in 4 cups of warm lukewarm water. Incorporate 1/4 cup apple cider vinegar or juice of a small lemon to help reduce the smell.

OCoconut oil is fantastic for skin care. It has the highest levels of caprylic acids, which is able to destroy Candida cells. Coconut oil is so gentle that it can be applied directly on your skin and nails. It can also be used to replace chemical-based creams and lotions.

To apply: gently to the affected areas after drying off and bathing. Apply until you take your next bath, or apply according to your preference. Massage coconut oil over feet and hands to stop fungal growth.

Take note: Always purchase top quality coconut oil, which is food grade. Avoid products with hydrogenation and partially hydrogenated coconut oils. These are contaminated with harmful solvents, such as Hexane, which can further damage tissues. It is not recommended for those suffering from or similar coconut (or similar) allergies.

Alternatives that have similar healing capabilities are:

SSAvocado oil

SSFlax (seed) oil

SSMacadamia oil

SSOlive oil, high-quality however, it doesn't have to be extra virgin.

SSPalm oil (not palm oil that is red as it stains skin)

SSPeanut oil

OGarlic is a rich source of allicin, which is naturally an antifungal as well as anti-microbial. Apply only to nails that are not broken. Rub garlic-based rubs to freshly cleaned skin. Let it sit for between 15 and 20 mins. Rinse thoroughly with antifungal soap. Apply a dry pat on the affected area using fresh paper towels. Use as often as you can. Use:

Equal parts of finely grated garlic minced and minced Epsom salt (use only for nails and skin that's not broken)

SS1 level tsp. of minced garlic, and 2 Tbsps. of olive oil

SS1 level tsp. of minced garlic, and 2 teaspoons. from white wine vinegar.

oHoney contains antibacterial and anti-inflammatory properties, as well as antifungal and antiseptic characteristics. It reduces the itchiness and irritation. This stops microorganisms reproducing and multiplying.

With a dropper of medicine use a dropper to apply a drop two drops of honey that is good quality at the base of the nail or on the areas that are affected. Allow the honey to air dry completely. Allow as long as is possible. It's safe even on split or broken nails as well as skin.

There is no reason to worry about getting ants or getting stung from insects when you apply honey. Honey of good quality is a great insect repellent due to its antiseptic strength.

Honey of poor quality is created of (or blended with) sugar that has been dissolved and then melted. The honey will draw insects.

To check its quality To test its quality, put a drop of it anywhere on the surface (e.g. countertop in the kitchen, or on the flooring) and let it sit for at least an hour. If insects are abounding on in the liquid amber, don't apply this to home remedies.

OLavender oil contains antifungal properties and is a popular treatment for cases of mild nail fungus.

To bathe: wash thoroughly prior to bed. Dry affected areas using an unclean towel or a wad of towels. Use a couple of drops lavender oil to the affected nails and the skin. Rub the oil on the fingertips. Apply the oil until you awake, or after 6 to 10 hours.

Combine equal amounts of lavender oil, the tea tree oil. A few drops of the oil can be applied of the oil to the affected skin and nails. Rub the oil with fingertips.

Do this every night or until nails start growing out. Utilize the same method as a preventive measure , at every week, at least after growth of nails that are healthier.

Be aware that this is not advised for severe or prolonged nail fungus infections. Always purchase therapeutic grade essential oils for treatment.

OLemon juice and lime juice which is best freshly squeezed. The citrus fruits have antifungal and antiseptic properties. They also smell wonderful. Place a couple of drops on your nails and smooth skin. Apply for minimum 15 minutes. Rinse the area with warm water. After that, dry the area.

Rub the spent citrus or lime peels/rinds at the nail's bottom to encourage rapid growth. The oil on the smooth surface of the nail contain high levels of calcium as well as Vitamin C. They include beta carotene, folate, magnesium, and potassium. In addition, it contains anti-inflammatory properties which can help alleviate pain caused by polyarthritis as well as rheumatoid arthritis.

Be careful to rub your nails gently to avoid damaging your nails and skin.

You can also mix equal portions of lime or lemon juice with olive oil. Apply a gentle rub to the affected areas. Let it sit to rest for the longest time is possible. Rinse gently. Pat-dry afterwards. This step should be done at least every day.

Olive leaf extract contains antimicrobial and antifungal qualities. This is a very light oil that can apply directly to your nails, or even on broken skin. Apply a few drops to the affected areas. Massage gently. Allow to remain on as long as you can. Repeat this step at least every day.

Combine 3 drops of extract from olive leaves in 3 Tbsps. Freshly squeezed lemon juice. Apply a few drops to nails and skin that isn't broken. Massage gently. Keep it on for as long as you can. Repeat this step at least each day. This will help eliminate unpleasant odors from affected areas.

OOrange oil contains antifungal properties which is employed to treat infections that are superficial.

To use: wash the affected region using a fresh cotton ball that is soaked in rub (ethyl) alcohol. Or in the event of breaks and cracks in the skin, cleanse the area using mild detergent and water. Dry with clean tissue paper.

Mix equal amounts of orange oil and any other mild carrier oil (e.g. olive oil or almonds.) Apply directly to the affected area(s) and let it sit for at least an hour. Apply a towel to dry the area if required. Repeat this step every day until the nails are grown out.

Make use of the same treatment as a preventive measure at minimum once per week after the growth of nails that are healthier.

Be aware that this is not advised for people who have sensitive skin or who are allergic to citrus-based oils. Always purchase therapeutic-grade essential oils to help with your skin issues.

Oregano oil has antifungal qualities.

To use: wash the affected area with an unclean cotton ball that has been which has been submerged in rub (ethyl) alcohol. Let the area air dry before proceeding.

Make 2 drops of oil from oregano per 20 drops of the mildest carrier oil (e.g. olive oil or almond oil.) Mix thoroughly. Put a small amount of the mixture onto an unclean cotton ball and gently apply it to the affected areas. Keep them on as long as is possible. Repeat the process three times a day until the nails have grown out.

Apply the same remedy as a preventive measure, at least every week following the regrowth of nails that are healthier.

Always purchase therapeutic-grade essential oils to use this home remedy, or , better yet make your own mix. (Recipe below.)

Solar Infused Oregano Oil Recipe

Put 1/2 cup of dried oregano along with 3/4 cup olive oil in a size Mason jar. Be sure the herbs are submerged. Use more oil only when necessary. You should ensure that there is at minimum an inch or two of headroom to allow the herbs to grow.

The jar is sealed with cling tape before fixing the lid. Set the jar in the direct sun (but away from humidity) for four to six weeks. Shake jar once a day to distribute oregano essence.

With a cheesecloth draped over colander or strainer, squeeze out the oregano. Make a knot with cheesecloth and squeeze as as much oil from the herb as is possible. Discard the herbs that are not used. Put oregano oil in a different Mason Jar. Secure lid. Utilize as required. Store in a cool, dark place (e.g. in a pantry or cabinet.) This can be stored for up to one year.

OTea tree oil contains antifungal and antiseptic qualities. It is a popular remedy for dermatophyte-related infections, particularly onychomycosis.

To clean the affected region using a fresh cotton ball that has been soaked in rub (ethyl) alcohol. Or If there are tears and cracks in the skin, clean the area using gentle detergent and water. Pat dry with dry, clean towelettes.

Mix equal parts from tea tree oils and any light carrier oil (e.g. olive oil or almond oil.) Apply directly onto the affected area(s) and allow to sit for at least 10 minutes. Utilizing a soft bristle toothbrush or nail file, rub the the area gently to eliminate the visible growth of fungal as is possible. Get rid of debris using clean towels. Repeat the process every day until nails get bigger.

Apply the same remedy as a preventive measure, at least every week following the growth of healthy nails.

You can also add some drops of tea tree oil along with some drops of peppermint oil to a bowl that is half filled with water. Soak your feet or hands for 20 minutes, then repeat the process twice every day for 20 minutes. Dry your feet and hands after each soak. This reduces reddening, pain and/or swelling.

Always purchase therapeutic-grade essential oils to treat ailments.

Combination with therapeutic oil. To mix the oils in a suitable container. In a bowl, dip a ball of cotton into and then hold it against the an affected area(s) for minimum three minutes. Let the area air dry. Repeat daily until nails have grown out.

SSAloe Vera gel (1 Tbsp.) along with tea tree oils (2 1 Tbsp.)

SSBasil oil, Tea tree oil (3 drops of each) combined together with coconut oil (1 Tbsp.)

SSCamphor oil (2 drops,) coconut oil (4 Tbsp.) along with Tea tree oil (3 drops)

Coconut oil Oregano oil, garlic peppermint oil, as well as Tea oil from the tree oil(3 drops per)

Oil SSCoconut (1/2 teaspoon.) as well as Neem oil (1/2 teaspoon.) as well as Tea tree oil (1 1 tsp.)

Oil SSCoconut (1/2 teaspoon.) as well as the oil of orange (1 1/2 teaspoon.) as well as the tea tree oil (1 teaspoon.)

SSCoconut oil (1 1 teaspoon.) along with tea tree oils (1 1 tsp.)

SSCoconut oil (1 1 tsp.), oregano oil (1/2 tsp.) and Tea tree oil (1 1 teaspoon.)

The oil is SSGrape (1/2 teaspoon.) as well as citrus oil (half a teaspoon.) as well as the tea tree oil (1 teaspoon.)

SSLavender oil (1 1 tsp.) along with tea tree oils (1 1 tsp.)

Oil SSMustard (1 2 Tbsp.) as well as Tea tree oils (3 drops)

Extract of SSOlive leaves (1 1 tsp.) along with tea tree oils (1 1 tsp.)

SSOlive oil (1 teaspoon.) along with tea tree oils (1 1 teaspoon.)

* Oral or internal home cures

Consume one tablespoon apple cider vinegar following each meal add 1 teaspoon of it with 1-cup of water that is warm. Make a alternative to afternoon or morning tea or coffee.

A regular intake of small quantities in apple cider vinegar not just help digestion to go quicker, but also boosts immunity. This keeps inflammation and infections at lower levels. It also speeds up healing.

Consume at least one portion of biotin-rich foods daily. Vitamin B7, also known as biotin, boosts metabolism and helps to limit the spread and growth of candida. This is a crucial nutritional ingredient to help maintain and speed up your growth rate of healthful skin, hair and nails.

Biotin-rich foods include:

SSAlmonds

SSBarley

Black-eyed peas from SSBlack-eyed Peas

The chicken liver and SSChicken

SSDairy

SSEdamame as well as soy beans and tofu

SSEggs

SSKidney beans

SSMushrooms

SSOats

Peanut butter and SSPeanuts

SSSalmon

SSTuna

SSWheat

Take a tablespoon of high honey of high-quality early in the day. usually prior to eating breakfast or the first drinks throughout the day. It boosts your immunity and reduces pain caused by inflammation.

It is advised for diabetics or those who are trying to regulate their insulin or blood sugar levels.

Add to your diet plain unflavored, plain yogurt that is not flavored. Yogurt is known for its beneficial quantities of microflora (probiotics) that contribute for gut health, however they also help keep parasites like microbes and fungi at bay.

Although consuming a small pot of yogurt (unsweetened/unflavored yogurt (between 125 grams to 150 grams) everyday will not cure nail fungus or fungal infection on its own, it will slow down fungal infestation. It is recommended to make use of it in conjunction alongside other home remedies or treatments.

It is suggested for lactose-intolerant individuals.

Other alternatives to yogurt that contain probiotics are: (NSFLIP = not suitable for lactose-intolerant persons)

SSBeet Kvass, at a minimum 1/2 cup per day

SSButtermilk homemade or traditional, (not commercial/cultured buttermilk,) at most 1/2 cup daily. NSFLIP

SSCheeses that are made from live cultures and high in probiotics. At least 1 Tbsp. daily, NSFLIP, specifically:

* Brick cheese

* Caciocavallo

* Cottage cheese

* Cheddar

* Edam

* Emmental

* Feta

* Gouda

* Gruyere

* Mozzarella

• Raw and unpasteurized and raw cow or goat cheeses

SSFermented ginger ale homemade, sugar-free and made from scratch, with at minimum 1 cup per day

SSGreen peas. At minimum 1/4 cup per day

SSMilk kefir at least one cup per day, NSFLIP

SSKimchi is recommended to consume at most 1/2 cup daily

SSKombucha or fermented tea at least one cup per day

SSMiso minimum 1 heaping tablespoon. per day. This condiment is great to mix into stews and soups.

SSNatto, at minimum 1/4 cup per day

SSPickles, most likely homemade minimum 1/4 cup per day

SSSauerkraut, at minimum 1 cup daily

SSTempeh At minimum 1/2 cup a day

SSUmeboshi or plums picked, at least one small piece each day

SSWater Kefir, at least 1 cup per day

Medicines and prescription medications such as.

The treatments must be prescribed by a healthcare professional. While many of them have been proved to be efficient against nail fungi as well as fungal infections, they may also have serious side effects.

A lot of them aren't suggested for children who are younger than 16 pregnant or lactating mothers, as well as patients with medical conditions such as diabetes or heart diseases.

It is highly recommended that you consult a physician prior to prescribing medication. Don't self-medicate if you're already taking another treatment (e.g. chemotherapy) or have had surgery, or are taking high-dose medications for other medical ailments.

* Oral medication. They are usually prescribed along in conjunction with other

medications. For moderate to severe cases of fungal nail fungus or nail infection, these medications are advised with topical application.

Antibiotics are typically prescribed in cases of chronic inflammation and infection are forming. They are usually prescribed along in conjunction with other medications.

OLamisil capsules or tablets aid in fighting infections caused by fungal infection. A daily dose can last from 6-12 weeks. It should not be done for individuals who have a compromised liver function.

Itraconazole capsules, capsules or tablets perform the same way as Lamisil (see earlier.)

* Over-the-counter treatments. While these are not prescription-based options but it is still advised that you seek the advice of your doctor before applying these.

oAlcohol-based mouthwash. It is known for its antiseptic and antibiotic properties, these mouthwashes may reduce the growth of fungal organisms. Apply only to areas of skin that are not broken.

To apply: pour a tiny bottles of mouthwash inside a smaller basin. Soak the affected areas in undiluted mouthwash in 15-20 mins. Dry the area afterward. Repeat once daily.

Pour a the mouthwash in a small bottle, together with half cup coconut vinegar and the juice of one small lime or lemon into a small bowl. Incorporate the lemons and lime wedges. Soak affected areas for between 15 and 20 minutes. Rinse thoroughly. Then, pat dry the area. Repeat once daily.

Antibacterial soaps. These soaps are typically employed to stop from spreading of fungal infections as well as other microbes. However, they do not treat nail fungus and fungal infections on their own.

OMedicated nail cream. Apply this cream to nails that are in pain following washing or soaking. Only use according to directions.

OMedicated nail polish especially penlac (ciclopirox). Paint a thin layer of it on the nails that are infected once per day for one week. Then, peel off the layers. Repeat the process each week for at least one year, or until the nails appear clear and glossy.

oVapor rubs. The application of vapor rubs on lightly affected areas will slow down the growth of fungal organisms and could stop the spread across the body. The high concentration of liniment reduces odors but does not eliminate them completely.

To use: clean affected areas with cleansing soap and water. Dry the area with dry, clean towels. Apply small dabs of lotion, but don't apply to damaged or broken skin. Apply until the next bath or wash the following day. Apply it once a day for at least three weeks.

OVitamin E oil can improve the health of the skin and nails. It has a high antioxidant capacity.

To use: puncture the capsule with a tiny vitamin and then apply some drops directly onto recently cleansed afflicted areas or areas with splintered or broken skin. Apply the longest time you can. Repeat this step at least every day.

* Topical or medicated Ointments. Apply only on the advice of your healthcare

provider particularly when you are taking prescription medicines or following any surgical procedure. Certain people experience extreme allergies to the drugs substances, which can lead to an increase in skin-related conditions.

oCicloprox-based cream. It is a well-known treatment for ringworms. It does not cause any adverse side negative effects. Take it as often as you need to.

oClotrimazol-based cream. This is a typical treatment for tinea, however it is not as effective against Dermatophytes. Make sure to use only according to the directions.

oEconazole-based cream. This is a typical treatment for tinea and is safe for use with no side consequences. Apply as required.

oEfinaconazole-based ointment. It's a powerful ingredient that is often utilized in cases of moderate to severe of fungal infections in the toes. This is less effective at eliminating tinea. Only use as directed.

oKetoconazole-based cream. It works by weakening the cellular walls of the fungi and preventing them from maturing properly and reproducing. A small amount is spread on the an affected region.

oLuliconazole-based cream. It is a popular treatment for tinea but it is not very effective against Dermatophytes. Only use according to the directions.

oMiconazole-based cream. It is a popular cure for yeast infection in vaginal vagina however you can also use it for treating tinea as well. Make sure to use it only as directed.

oMiranel cream. It contains the same ingredients that are found in most steam rubs but is infused with tea tree oil and miconazole, a antifungal, Nitrate. Apply it on freshly cleaned skin, especially at evening. Keep it on for at the minimum 8 hours a day.

oNaftifine-based cream. It is a popular treatment for tinea and also moderately effective against Dermatophytes. Only use according to the directions.

oOxiconazole-based cream. It is particularly effective against dermatophytes that can cause onychomycosis. Make sure to use only as directed.

oTavaborole-based ointment. It is a different ingredient utilized for moderate to advanced cases of fungal infections in the toe. Make sure to use only as directed.

oTerninafine-based cream. This cream is especially effective against dermatophytes that can cause onychomycosis. This reduces reddening, itching and swelling of the affected areas. Only use according to the directions.

Cream containing oUndecylenic acid. This cream is especially effective against dermatophytes causing onychomycosis. Apply as required.

* Other types of treatment

OLaser treatment. As of 2015, medical specialists claimed that laser therapy can eradicate nail fungus caused by Dermatophytes (onychomycosis.) This is however an indefinite, and quite costly treatment. It is only available upon the advice of an dermatologist.

The removal of nails surgically. This is an extremely extreme step to getting rid of nail fungus. After the nail is removed applying topical treatments directly to the skin until the nails grow and grow back.

Food therapy. Much like Chinese tradition, certain foods can help improve
health. However, they should be utilized in conjunction with other treatments alternatives.

For instance, supplement your every day by taking Vitamin E capsules or other food items that are rich in this nutrient, for example, as:

SSAlmonds

Nectarines, SSApricots, and peaches

SSAsparagus

SSAvocadoes

SSBasil

The peppers of SSBell

SSBlackberries and raspberries

SSBroccoli

SSButternut squash

SSChili powder

SSCollards

SSCrayfish and lobsters

SSGreen olives

SSGuavas

SSHazelnuts

SSHerring

SSKale

SSKiwi fruit

SSMamey Sapote

SSMangoes

SSMulberries

SSMustard greens

SSOlive oil

SSOregano

SSOysters

SSPaprika

SSParsley

SSPeanuts

SSPecans

SSPine nuts

SSPistachio nuts

SSPumpkin seeds

SSRainbow trout

SSSalmon

Shrimps and SSShrimps

SSSesame seeds

SSSpinach

Seeds of squash and SSSquash

SSSunflower seeds

SSSwiss the chard

SSSwordfish

SSTomatoes

SSTurnip greens

SSWalnuts

Consume foods and drinks which boost the immune system, such as:

SSApple

SSAvocado

SSBanana

SSBeef

Peppers from SSBell

Blueberry cherries, chokeberry Goji berry and cranberry grapes and strawberry

SSGreen tea and black tea

SSBroccoli

SSBrussels sprouts

SSChicken and turkey

SSCitruses, more specifically: Clementine, grapefruit, lemon lime, orange and Tangerine

SSDried fruits, particularly raisins and sultanas

SSFatty fish, in particular mackerel, herring tuna, and salmon

SSGarlic

SSGinger and turmeric

SSKale

SSKiwi fruit

SSMangosteen

SSMushrooms, dried or fresh specifically: maitake Reishi, and Shiitake

SSNuts, specifically hazelnuts, pecans and almonds and walnuts

SSOats and barley

SSPapaya

SSPear

SSPomegranate

SSPumpkin and squash

The SSShellfish include lobsters, crabs and clams as well as oysters, mussels and clams.

SSSpinach

SSSunflower seeds

SSSweet potato

SSYogurt

Chapter 14 Supplements

The body performs optimally in the presence of everything that it requires to look after its own needs. This is also true with regards to the body's fight against infection and the overgrowth of fungus. Supplements can be used as an additional layer for providing the body with the necessary nutrients.

Grapefruit Seed Extract

Extract of grapefruit is derived of the membranes, seeds and grapefruit pulp. It is extremely effective in fighting infections and is antifungal in nature. It can be consumed in capsules or liquid form. The liquid form may be applied directly to the toenail and surrounding skin. It is also used as an antiseptic to keep the feet free of fungal infection.

According to 'Benefits of Grapefruit Seed Extract', an article by Tamara Jankoski at 'Applied Health' (http://appliedhealth.com/benefits-of-grapefruit-seed-extract/), studies completed by Dr. J.A. Botino of the University of So Paulo in Brazil Grapefruit seeds have been found that it is 100% effective in cleaning the skin prior to surgery, when compared to 72% efficacy that alcohol has and 98% efficacy for surgical soaps when used in a scrub application for one minute.

Vitamin C

Anything that improves the resistance to infection can help in preventing the occurrence of toenail fungus infection. Vitamin C is typically linked to helping your body to fight off colds, however, it can also be beneficial in preventing infections as well as to speed up the healing process for existing infections. If you're susceptible to infections of the toenails, taking an everyday vitamin C supplement could be the solution you require. Choose a high-quality product that does not contain additives. You can take the vitamin in amounts of up to 500 mg each at least three or four every day because the body is able to absorb around 500 mg per day. Vitamin C is water-soluble and any excess amount will be excreted through urine.

Probiotics

If you've been following health-related news in the last few years, you've likely heard lots of probiotics-related information. Probiotics are a group of bacteria which line the digestive tract. They are vital to maintaining healthy living because they aid the body in a variety of ways, including helping maintain its capacity to take in nutrients that are absorbed from foods. The reason why probiotics are crucial for people susceptible to fungus that affects the toenails is because they assist the body fight infections and eliminate the overabundance of harmful bacteria and fungi which can cause harm to the body.

In the next section within this chapter, you can consume probiotic foods like yogurt or kefir, fermented veggies sauerkraut, and other fermented vegetables. If you're not a fan of eating these kinds of foods, even if it's just at least once a week, taking probiotic supplements could be a better choice for you to help keep the gut bacteria in check and maintain it to prevent the growth of harmful fungal strains.

There are numerous probiotic supplements available and not all probiotics are made in the same way. You should choose the right probiotic to combat infection. Find a reputable brand that has a greater number of probiotics ranging from between 15 and 100 billion, as well as one with between 10 and 30 strains. Probiotics are available in a variety of supplement stores as well as health food stores that sell supplements and vitamins.

Zinc

Consuming 50 milligrams of zinc every day is another method to strengthen your immune system fight off the fungi that are responsible for toenail fungus.

Goldenseal Herb

Goldenseal has been shown in numerous studies to be an effective natural antibiotic that doesn't cause any adverse unwanted side negative effects. Use the daily dose of goldenseal according to the brand you purchase in tincture or capsule form.

Surgery

A Surgery Alternative:

Many who are suffering from frequent toenail fungus infections might want to eliminate the toenail in order to not have to worry about the ongoing possibility of the fungus coming back and needing to go through the lengthy process of treatment again.

During the procedure it is possible for the entire nail to be removed, or a portion of the nail may be removed, based on how infected the fungal infection has become, however, if the aim is to prevent any further infections when the nail has grown back in the future, the nail matrix has to be destroyed with the help of a chemical, such as phenol to the cuticle region. Otherwise, the body will take the natural course and create a new nail. The straightforward procedure is performed at the physician's office, and an antibiotic can be used for a few weeks following the procedure. The procedure is reasonably affordable and not too strenuous.

This is the Laser Treatment Alternative:

The most recent treatment for fungus of the toenails is laser therapy. There are a variety of laser therapy to treat nail fungus. Sometimes, the treatment with lasers is utilized in conjunction with other medications. The way in which the laser treatment works is lasers generate the energy of light and heat which damages the tissue in just the area of focus, but without damaging the surrounding tissue. Another benefit of laser therapy is that the amount of time invested is extremely minimal and there isn't any time to recover.

Laser treatments are not usually insured as they are considered to be an alternative treatment, and are costly. Laser treatments can be a boon in the medical field and there was a Food and Drug Administration approved treatments using lasers for nail fungus only a couple of years in the past, based on research published in medical journals, experts have said that there aren't enough blinded studies of comparison that include enough patients to determine whether or not laser treatments are effective in the treatment of nail fungus. If you think that laser therapy could be an option for you, speak to your physician about it.

Chapter 15: Nail Fungus Traditional Treatment Options

It is the first thing to begin by having an examination with a family physician or general practitioner. If your doctor refers youto a specialist, you can be examined immediately by dermatologist (skin specialist) or a podiatrist (foot specialist). An accurate diagnosis is crucial since the fungus could mimic other conditions like psoriasis. It is necessary to gather details for your doctor to ensure that an accurate report is made and a plan for treatment is set.

Appointment Preparation

It is crucial to be prepared before you see to see your physician for your first visit. When you aren't carrying medical records that you can transfer, you'll have to make arrangements with the following:

Step 1: Create your list of symptoms, including any information that may not be related to the nail fungus.

Step 2: Create your own list of all your personal details. Make sure you include any life-changing events that have occurred recently or other major stress-related issues you might be experiencing at the moment.

Step 3: Compile a list of each of our medications--vitamins--or other supplements should also be listed.

Step 4: Create an inventory of all the questions you'll have to ask the doctor.

Questions to ask

Here are a few questions you need to ask about the nail fungus

Question 1: Are there other possible causes for the symptoms and condition?

Question 2. Is there a most probable cause for the symptoms and condition?

Question 3: What tests are needed?

4. Are there alternatives to the strategy you're suggesting?

Question 5: What's the most efficient method of action?

6. I have additional health issues. How do I deal with both simultaneously?

Question 7 Would you like to know whether you can find an equivalent generic medicine for this new medication?

Question 8 Do you have informational materials, either on the internet or in brochures that I could bring at home?

It is crucial to be fully prepared when you arrive at the appointment.

Diagnostics and Tests

It is the first thing to get your nails examined. The doctor can collect a sample by scraping a small amount of dirt off the nail bed or by drilling a tiny hole into the nail. The nail will then send to a laboratory to determine the kind of fungus that is causing the disease.

It is crucial to conduct an exam to determine the cause of your nail as other conditions, such as psoriasis could cause the same fungal infection to your nail. Finding out the root cause can provide the solution for the most effective option for treatment. It is estimated that around 50- sixty percent cases of the appearance of the nail resulted from the fungus.

Certain insurers require lab test to determine if the antifungal medication is included on an insurance claim. The nail will be cultivated or stained through PCR (Polymerase Chain Reaction) to determine the genetic material that makes up the organism. The staining process and the culture is about six weeks long, but fungal identification can be accomplished in just one day.

The Treatments of Your Physician

Based on how severe the infection has gotten; you may require an array of medicines to treat the fungal infection. The first medications that are used:

Gels, creams or lotions that are applied directly to nails

Lacquer for nails that is applied to the surface

An antifungal oral prescription medication (pill)

Removal of the damaged part of the nail or skin

It is crucial to monitor closely due to the possibility of adverse negative side effects. In the event of a severe infection, depending on the nail infection is the nail may require removal surgically. Topical medicines are typically utilized for moderate-to-moderate infections. For instance, you could stop the spread of athlete's foot to the nail, or suffer an infection recur if you don't treat it with Ointments.

Nail cream containing Medicated Nail Cream

After soaking, apply an antifungal lotion prescribed by your physician to the nails that are infected. The cream is most effective by first thinning the nails so that the medication can penetrate the hard nail surface.

Then thin the nails: It is necessary to buy a non-prescription, over-the-counter lotion that contains urea. Your doctor can also thin the nail's surface using the file for nails or other device.

Nail Lacquer/Nail Paint

The oral route has more efficacy, however your physician will inform you on the best option suitable for the specific kind of disease.

Amorolfine (Loceryl) is an ingredient that's active in nail lacquer, which is an antifungal medicines and is a suitable alternative to the majority (not all) types of nail-related infections. The lacquer can be purchased in pharmacies, and also with an appointment.

The lacquer can be useful toward the nail's end. But, it won't perform as well when there is an nail infection that is near the skin or the skin surrounding the nail.

Follow the instructions precisely in applying nail varnish in order to get the greatest chances of success. It can take as long as six months to repair your fingernails, or up to a year for toenails.

Ciclopirox topical solution 8 percent (Penlac) It is an medical nail lacquer that has been approved to treat of the fingernail or toenail that does not involve the lunula (white part that is the white portion of nails) and specifically for those who have healthy immune systems. The product has a success rate of 7% percent when applied on nails on a daily basis for up an entire year. As of the moment, 2016--the product is unavailable on the market in the United States.

Fluconazole (Diflucan) Fluconazole (Diflucan) medication is given for a period of time and may be administered one time every week. The dosage may require adjustment when a patient is on other medications, or if the patient has impaired liver function or kidney disease. It's not as efficient in the same way as Sporanox and Lamisil.

Notification: A blood test can detect liver disease.

Medicines

In certain instances the antifungal tablets can eliminate fungal nail infections and can also treat other skin diseases like athlete's foot.

Itraconazole Tablets (Sporanox): This is a pulsed therapy. Adults must take 200 mg every day for a week, and then repeat the course after 21 days have passed. Toenails require at least three sessions, while fingernails could only require two courses.

Terbinafine Tablets (Lamisil) Terbinafine Tablets (Lamisil) dosage for adults daily of 250 mg. For fingernails the treatment is required for six weeks between three and six months. Toenails: The treatment is required for 3 to 6 months. Signs of improvement should be evident within two months for fingernails and after three months for healthier toenails.

Tavaborole Topical (Kerydin) Tavaborole Topical (Kerydin) medication is brand new in the marketplace as an antifungal oxaborole product. It is indicated for the treatment of onychomycosis in the toenail only. It is recommended to apply it each day for at least for 48 weeks. Avoid using close to your mouth, eyes or in your vagina.

Ticonazole: This drug is also applied to nails and is prescribed. It has been proven to not perform as well as amorolfine.

Efinaconazole (Jublia) It is a medicine was approved by the FDA in 2014. It is an ointment for topical use applied on the skin to treat toenail mentagrophytes of

Trichophyton as well as Trichophyton rubrum. It should apply to the affected area every day for up to 48 weeks.

Griseofulvin (Gris-Peg, Gifulvin, and Fulvicin) The medication is available in tablet, liquid or capsule forms and typically taken daily however, it can be used up to four times per throughout the day. The medication should be carefully controlled and has a variety of risks. Stay under the supervision of a doctor during the course of this medication that must be used for up to one year to heal nail infection. This treatment treats nail discoloration.

Ketoconazole (Buzirak) Ketoconazole (Buzirak) is an effective oral treatment for candida fungus or if the yeast does not respond to griseofulvin. The medication is available regularly and is monitored by a doctor. There are some adverse negative effects. Some doctors aren't recommending the use of it due to its numerous side effects and interactions with other drugs.

Research has confirmed that five out of ten patients that are treated for fungal infections appear normal. However, two of 10 cases will be cleared of the fungus, however the nail will never look normal for the rest of its life. For those who are over 65 years old older, the chances of success could be lower. Combining oral and topical treatments improves the outcomes.

The reasons for failure Fingernails are known to respond better to treatments. Sometimes, treatments fail because the medication is taken off too fast. It is essential to adhere to the instructions given by your doctor as well as research proven to treat nail fungus infection.

Side Effects: Like every treatment you take, it is possible that you may be confronted with issues that range from rashes to damage to your liver.

Lasers and Light-Based Therapies

Different types of laser treatments:

The following are the boundaries of the wavelengths used in laser treatments:

660 nanometers (nm) visible light in red

940 nm near-infrared light

1064 nm neodymium-doped yttrium aluminum garnet laser (Nd:YAG)

This NdYAG laser is typically one that is pumped, which makes use of diodes for lasers of flash lamps to generate energy within the wavelength 1064nm.

Laser Treatment The Method

The laser is used to shine the targeted, soft light beam onto the nails and skin. The laser shines on the nail to kill embedded fungus on the nail plate or bed where the fungus dwells.

This technique requires more research However, when used in conjunction in conjunction with medication, the light can help your nails improve. One study of 24 individuals found benefits of a carbon dioxide laser therapy treatment program that included an antifungal cream for nails.

Anesthesia is not required for laser treatments. If you feel any discomfort during the treatment, the laser's power is reduced. Certain people may experience occasional snapping sensation or a slight heat throughout the procedure, however generally speaking, there hasn't been any post-treatment discomfort observed.

The treatment with lasers for your nails is typically going to be 30 minutes long to finish. The majority of clinical studies indicate that the first treatment will result in an improvement in your nails.

Be aware that some insurance companies aren't willing to be able to cover the procedure as it's considered to be cosmetic. These procedures are expensive and not available in every area.

Laser therapy has been proven to be effective, with a low rate of recurrence of the infection for up to five years after treatment. Laser therapy is advantageous since you will not experience any medication-related side effects.

(PDT) or Photodynamic Therapy (PDT)

This treatment relies on an molecule that can be triggered by light. normally activated by a substance that is activated by lighting. The procedure can be carried out in an outpatient facility like a doctor's office. Three steps are required:

Step 1. A light-sensitizing lotion liquid or intravenous substance (photosensitizer) is used or applied.

Step 2: A period of incubation can be expected between minutes and days.

3. The target nail or tissue is exposed to light wavelength that activates the medication that is photosensitive.

PDT is used currently in a variety of medical areas, including cosmetic surgery and oncology.

Ultrasound

Low-frequency ultrasound can enhance the permeability of an infected nail. If you apply the ultrasound therapy onto the nail it allows pits to develop and more topical medication can be delivered. Software interfaces provide the capability to choose the toes to be treated, and provides an intensity level that is low, medium or high.

Create Holey Nails

Harvard team of researchers is finding ways to treat toe fungus by providing the most direct path to the root of the fungus. Through cutting holes into the nail, doctors can treat beneath the nail. But, do not try this at your home!

The trickiest part of the procedure that restricts the patient's capacity to perform the act is to make the holes sufficiently deep. After the hole has been made then antifungal cream is inserted inside the holes. But, it is important to be aware of the procedure in case you push too far it could pierce the soft tissue containing nerves underneath the nail.

Technology has improved, so the latest instrument that has sensors can sense the change in resistance and determine when it is time to stop drilling. However most insurance companies view the procedure to be cosmetic and won't pay for it.

You can receive coverage for diabetes as the fungus could be extremely harmful and cause numerous other illnesses.

Removal of Nails

The application of a local anesthetic can be used to remove the nail after the other treatment options have not worked. It could be the only alternative for treatment in case the nail is extremely painful. The new nail will grow in slowly, however it may take a while. Following removal, treatment will consist of antifungal medicine.

However, a total cure, which is defined as clinical cure (implying clearing of the nail) and mycological treatment (both negative microscopy and dermatophyte cultivation) is usually not possible.

Chemical Nail Removal

The removal of the nail by chemical is a non-invasive procedure to remove only the affected or diseased portion of the nail. The nail can be removed in two ways: a portion (debridement) as well as the whole (avulsion) nail is removed.

The process starts by applying a tape-like adhesive cloth over the skin that is not affected surrounding the nail. A urea ointment is sprayed on the top of the nail and protected by tape and plastic. Within seven to ten weeks, the ointment softens the nail. The dressing needs to remain dry.

If you visit the office of a doctor The nail will be removed and removed from its nail bed and the affected area is removed.

The area needs to remain dry for a further two weeks. It will be healed within that time. Toenails can take anywhere from 12 to 18 months to grow again. Fingernails typically grow back in six months.

This procedure can be applied on nails that have increased in size due to hypertrophic (abnormal growth) as well as for serious antifungal infections.

Take note of using an antibiotic ointment to avoid infection. The fungal infection may not be completely eradicated and may be re-infected when it expands.

Chapter 16: What is Nail Fungus Cured?

Patience is the first on the list on the priority list for the question of how to treat nail fungus. These are the most important aspects:

Proper care of infected feet

If you suffer from an acute or mild fungal infection, or none at all, it's vital to look after your feet. This is the best way to reduce the chance of future outbreaks

Rinse your food with water and soap.

Dry your feet completely between your toes.

Straight across the toenails, making sure they are shorter than the tip of the toe.

Make sure you keep the files and clippers clean by washing them with water and soap. Wipe the tools clean using alcohol.

Do not paint your nails using polish. The nail bed can't breathe it', which could prevent the fungal growth from leaving the.

Conduct visual checks

It is crucial to conduct an annual check of your nail beds and skin surrounding your toenails. Make use of a mirror if can't see your nails clearly. Examine any changes in texture or color and also any cuts or injuries. If you observe any unusualities contact your physician for the information.

Select the Best Footwear

You must select suitable shoes made from the right material to let air flow through it, for example mesh or canvas. Use socks that remove moisture from your feet. Make sure you change them frequently. If you're in public spaces, like locker rooms or pools take the shower shoe as a precautionary step.

What to Look For In Treatment

The treatment will kill the fungus However, the nail will be left until it grows. A healthy, fresh nail will begin to develop at the base of the nail to prove that the treatment is effective. It could take a few months for the infected portion on the nail develop out and then be clipped.

The fingernails will get bigger faster. Don't be discouraged since you might wait a whole year until your toenails are normal. After a few months of therapy, you'll be able to see some growth. If you don't, consult with your physician. The infection could being responding to therapy as the medication used to treat the fungal infection remains within the nail about nine months after treatment is finished.

Select the Plan

Oral medications (antifungal pills) gives you the greatest chances of curing fungal infections. Unfortunately, there are some who experience adverse consequences. The use of antifungal pills is usually for cases of moderate or severe of fungal nail infections.

Antifungal topical remedies like gels, lacquers or creams, are applied to adjacent areas of the nail and directly on the nail. Although they may not be as effective as oral medications however, they are generally not associated with any lasting adverse consequences. Most often, topical medicines are most effective for moderate to mild illnesses.

You Must Choose

It is important to consider the type of infection you are suffering from as well as the potential side effects and the price of the treatment you select.

Chapter 17: Nail Fungus Natural Treatment Options

There are many kinds of natural treatments and remedies are available; some can be are available within your home.

White Vinegar

Mix 1 part White Vinegar and 2 parts warm water.

Soak the affected area for 10 to 15 minutes.

Rinse the area to stop the fungus spreading.

Dry completely.

Repeat the process each day.

Be sure to add more liquid to the mixture in case there is any sign of irritation.

Apple Cider Vinegar (ACV)

Mix equal amounts of apple cider vinegar in order to make the antifungal mix.

It is also possible to make the paste by mixing a few teaspoons of vinegar from apple cider as well as crushed rice flower. The paste can be applied and scrubbed directly onto the areas affected. The solution will also eliminate the dead cells of your skin.

Baking Soda and Vinegar

1 Cup White or Apple Cider Vinegar

4.5-2 Tablespoons Baking Soda

Water

Mix the Vinegar in enough water to bathe your feet.

For 15 minutes, soak in the tub.

Pat dry using paper towels.

Make sure to add several Tablespoons of Baking soda to water that is enough to bathe your feet.

Let it soak for about 15 mins.

Dry your feet using towelettes.

The vinegar kills the fungus and baking soda can stop development of nail.

This process should be done early in the morning, and later at the night.

Cayenne Pepper

Your body is able to better fight fungal infections if you include cayenne pepper in your food preparation. It is a great digestion and immune support that can boost your metabolism and circulation.

Honey

Honey is a common remedy to soothe sore throats, but it can also be beneficial as an anti-bacterial natural ingredient. Honey is a rich source of hydrogen peroxide, which is known to draw toxins out of your feet.

Add a teaspoon of honey on the toenail.

Cover the area affected with gauze.

It is also possible to take a teaspoon of vinegar from apple cider as well as 1 tablespoon honey for an everyday infection prevention.

Seeds of Pumpkin Seeds

Omega-3 fatty acids have a high in pumpkin seeds. They also have antiviral, antiparasitic and antifungal properties. Additionally, you will get an improvement in mood with higher intake of omega-3.

Salt

Get a salt bath! If you've got any open sores on your feet, the salt bath is exactly the thing you'll need.

Mix two Teaspoons of Salt in 1 quart of warm water.

Pour the mix into a shallow dish.

Relax your feet in the water for five to 10 minutes.

Repeat the procedure several times per throughout the day, until your infection has subsided.

Lemon Juice

The juice of a lemon contains citric acid that helps in stopping the spreading of fungus and bacteria infections. Place the juice of a freshly squeezed lemon directly to your nail and leave it for 10 mins. Rinse thoroughly with warm water. Repeat this process daily for about a month for optimal results.

Mustard Powder

The powder is loaded with a powerful acid that kills fungus.

1. Add one Teaspoon of Mustard Power to a shallow pan that is filled with warm water.

Soak your feet for about 30 minutes.

Repeat the procedure until the fungus goes away during the night and morning.

Apply the paste on each affected nail. You can also apply the paste on the athlete's feet. Cover your feet and foot with cellophane so that the past can't run. Keep the wrap on for at least 30 minutes, or for the entire day, if you want.

Be sure to wash and dry thoroughly your feet. Keep your towel away from the rest of your family. Don't let the fungus on the damp towel.

Yogurt

Yogurt is a food source that has a probiotic with nutrients that can speed up the healing process for fungus. (See the entire chapter in Chapter 8).)

Additional Treatments: Don't Believe

Baking Soda and Borax

The fungus requires an acidic environment to thrive, which makes baking soda that is alkaline a great solution to stop the fungus from flourishing. Borax/sodium borate is an organic mineral that also acts as an effective fungicide.

If the two ingredients are mixed in equal amounts of water to create an emulsion, you've got the quickest cure to treat nail fungus.

Soak your feet in water and gently rub the mixture on the nails that are infected.

Repeat this two times a day for at least two weeks following the time when the fungus seems to be gone.

Corn Meal

Corn naturally has a fungus form which is safe for the human body , but it is not a Candida--a popular fungal parasite that causes infections for many people. Make sure you use a large container to wash your feet or foot. Mix:

One Cup Corn Meal

Two Quarts of water

Let the mix be sat for at least an hour.

Submerge feet and feet within the vessel for at most half an hour or longer.

Make the mix as often as you like since it's completely natural.

Hydrogen Peroxide

Mix water and an equal mixture of hydrogen peroxide 3. For 18 to 20 minutes soak in this solution to ensure rapid healing of the fungal infection.

Listerine Mouthwash

Utilize a solution of Listerine or a similar kind of mouthwash mixed with vinegar and lemon juice. Make the mixture an infusion for between 10 and 15 minutes.

Rubbing Alcohol

Rub alcohol straight on your feet for some minutes of care. Dry your feet thoroughly.

Camphor and Vicks VapoRub

Camphor is created by distilling bark and wood of the Camphor Tree. Today, camphor is produced from turpentine and used for Vicks VapoRub.

Rubs are great to reduce itching and ease discomfort. It can also be helpful for fungal infections that affect the toenail. The camphor boosts local circulation of blood to the affected area , and also stimulates nerve endings. But, don't rub on the broken skin. It's a great product that can be used in a variety of ways.

Cut and cut the nail.

Rinse the area affected and then dry it completely.

Wrap the area in gauze or an elastic bandage.

Put on a pair of socks. Repeat the procedure every day. It could take between six and 10 weeks before it's fully healed However, it is likely to work.

Others have said that even they felt that Vicks cough syrup could aid in the process.

Clove Oil

Eugenol is also found in the clove oil. Clove can also be a great pain reliever, as the principal ingredient:

2 teaspoons olive Oil (optional) as well Coconut Oil

4 - 8 Drop Clove Oil

Mix the ingredients and apply the mixture to the toenails. If the skin is damaged you can weaken the oil by applying coconut oil or olive oil. It is possible to repeat the process twice to three times a day.

Coconut Oil

Caprylic acid can be described as a medium-chain fat acid that is found in coconut oil that can penetrate the hard cell wall of fungi. If the protective layer of the fungus becomes damaged and the cells break down, and the infection is cured.

Place a light layer oil on the affected areas and allow the solution to soak for approximately 15 minutes. It is possible to apply the oil since this is an organic ingredient. Be sure to check a small part of your face prior to applying the oil. apply the oil on your nail bed.

Garlic Oil

Make use of equal amounts of white vinegar and garlic oil to provide a natural treatment for the area affected. Apply the mixture over the area and then cover it with the elastic bandage. Allicin's properties are contained in garlic that has anti-fungal components. It is possible to substitute olive oil for crushed garlic if you do not have garlic oil. Each day, you should have an extra clove of garlic to protect yourself.

You can also use fresh garlic and cut into two halves (diagonally). Grate it on the nail's edge and push the pulp beneath the nail's edge. Utilize a toothpick to push the pulp into the bottom of your nail. It's not harmful and it will also paint the nail's surface with lacquer. Two weeks of application is reported to be successful.

Lavender Oil

Lavender is a natural antiseptic that has many properties that aid in home remedy for minor cases of fungus on the toes. Utilize a cotton ball to apply the oil on the surface of the nail infected. Put on a thick pair socks to allow the solution be more effective. If you apply this treatment over the course of a night and you are sure to get positive results.

When purchasing Lavender essential oil ensure that you're buying pure essential oil, not one that has fragrance added. The oil can be purchased in specific herbal stores, however it could be expensive.

Lemon Eucalyptus Oil

The oil is extracted of the lemon eucalyptus trees It can be applied to the skin for anti-fungal medicine. It doubles to repel insects.

Neem Oil

The neem plant produces the oil neem, which is indigenous to India and is a similarity to mahogany. People in India have been using the oil for years to treat a variety of fungus growths. This includes nail fungus. Neem is applied multiple times a day on the affected nails until the infection has gone away.

It is important to note that the usage of neem must be not be used during pregnancy or breastfeeding.The oil must also remain out of the reach for children due to the potential for Reye's syndrome-like symptoms. It can also cause death when consumed.

Olive Leaf Oil

The elimination of yeast from your body by the powerful antimicrobial properties of the olive leaf.

Orange Oil

Every day, you can apply one dropper of oil between your toes and beneath the toenails. The oil should be left to rest for around an hour. The oil that is orange can be mixed with a similar amount in any oil carrier.

Conclusion

It is often regarded as a minor problem nail fungus is often thought of as a minor issue. However, it may cause fungal infection that can cause other medical issues that are more serious. Do not take this illness lightly.

There are a variety of simple home remedies that can be followed to keep nail fungal infections at the bare minimum. This book provides treatments that use items you typically find in your pantry or cupboard. They include soaks, rubs and sprays made of natural ingredients such as coconut oil, baking soda and vinegar.

I hope this book will give you more information on how to treat nail fungus without resorting costly medicines or extreme surgical procedures. The book also offers preventive strategies and suggestions for taking care of your nails, hands and the skin generally to ensure that you are healthy and in top shape.

It is the next thing to do: locate some solutions at home (within this guidebook) which you can use to eliminate and prevent the recurrence of nail fungal growth. It is also suggested to test certain ingredients that are that are listed under "food for therapy."